Praise for *Menu for Life* from the Obesity Study participants:

"Thank you, Dr. Randall and Donna Randall for your combined wisdom, dedication, and determination to get this book done so that others will benefit from the Menu for Life philosophy. Participating in the Randalls' Menu for Life program at Howard University gave me a new lease on LIFE. Now, I am enjoying their book so much! In fact, I stayed up until 2:30 a.m. because I was reading with great interest. Already, I am feeling even more committed to continuing my Menu for Life. You have made such a contribution to society because you have written this book! Yesterday, when I went to church, I wore one of my dresses from 'my former petite life.' That dress is about sixteen years old but it doesn't look out of date because it has classic details. I decided I *will* wear that dress again. And I am!"

—MARIE PRIMAS-BRADSHAW

"Weighing over 350 pounds at age 38, with diabetes and high blood pressure, I had a massive stroke. I'm 48 years old now, and my weight is down to 200 pounds. My blood pressure is 120/80, and I don't take medication for hypertension, or for diabetes. Dr. Randall and Donna Randall gave us the tools in the Menu for Life program—Mrs. Randall can come and cook for me any time! But we have to live the program out for ourselves every day—keep to the front of the reality that is going on. My biggest mission—I pray on this every day—is that I can touch someone's life. I don't need to know who; I just want to help people make positive changes. Maybe it will be *you*. Read this book and let it change your life!"

—CEDRIC WILLIAMS

"All the participants in the Menu for Life study, every one of us, had overeaten until we were obese. When you do that, it causes all kinds of health problems and an early demise. I don't want to leave this Earth one second earlier than I have to! Dr. Randall and Donna Randall taught us about portion control, about how to eat less food, better food, and still keep ourselves full. After the program, you have a tendency to go back to the way you used to eat. But you should want to *live*, not *eat*. My motto now is to eat only when I'm hungry, eat till I'm satisfied, and stop when I'm full. Thank you Dr. Randall and Donna Randall!"

—STEPHANIE DOVE

Menu for Life

~~~~~~

African Americans
Get Healthy,
Eat Well,
Lose Weight,
and
Live Beautifully

OTELIO S. RANDALL, M.D.,
AND DONNA RANDALL

PRODUCED BY AMARANTH

Broadway Books   NEW YORK

BROADWAY BOOKS titles may be purchased for business or promotional use or for special sales. For information, please write to: Special Markets Department, Random House, Inc., 1745 Broadway, New York, New York 10019.

PRINTED IN THE UNITED STATES OF AMERICA

This book is not intended to take the place of medical advice from a trained medical professional. Readers are advised to consult a physician or other qualified health professional regarding treatment of their medical problems. Neither the publisher nor the author take any responsibility for any possible consequences from any treatment, action, or application of medicine, herb, or preparation to any person reading or following the information in this book.

BROADWAY BOOKS and its logo, a letter B bisected on the diagonal, are trademarks of Broadway Books, a division of Random House, Inc.

Visit our website at www.broadwaybooks.com

First edition published 2003.

Designed by Margaret M. Wagner

Illustrated by Simon M. Sullivan

Library of Congress Cataloging-in-Publication Data

Randall, Otelio Sye

Menu for life: African Americans get healthy, eat well, lose weight, and live beautifully / Otelio S. Randall and Donna Randall.

p.cm.

Includes index.

ISBN 0-7679-0993-3

1. Reducing diets. 2. Obesity—Treatment. 3. Weight loss. 4. African Americans—Health and hygiene. I. Randall, Donna II. Title.

RM222.2 R355 2003

613-25—dc21   2003034158

10 9 8 7 6 5 4 3 2 1

To the loving memory of my father, Oran Leo Rideout, whose spiritual guidelines continue to light my way. And to Momma, my children—Otelio II, Paula, Kari, and Cydnee, along with my brothers and sister—Wendell, Leo Jr., and Sharon, who between them managed to sample at one time or another every single morsel of my creations. Above all, to Him in whom we trust.

—DONNA RANDALL

To my parents, who devoted their lives to the education and welfare of their children. To my sisters—Bertrua, Greta and Jaycina, Clementine and Ella Mae (deceased) for their support, love, and friendship. To my brother Canoy, who meant everything to me. And to my children—Otelio II, Paula, Karintha, and Cydnee, for the thrills they have provided for Donna and me.

—OTELIO S. RANDALL, M.D.

Contents

~~~~~

Introduction

~~~~~~~

Where, and when, did our Menu for Life start? It is as difficult for Donna and for me to pinpoint its beginning as it is to envision where our Menu for Life will lead us. Although it just now comes to you as a book, *Menu for Life* was born long ago, even before our children, when our careers and our lives together were just beginning, when I was a young cardiologist fellow at the University of Michigan and Donna was acquiring a reputation as a gourmet cook. Sadly, it was the time when Donna lost her father to heart disease . . . and awakened to the harsh reality that she, too, had the start of the health problem that led to his death: high blood cholesterol.

When it became clear that Donna needed to change her eating habits to improve her health, she turned to the only answer she knew: cooking. Her interest in gourmet foods went back to childhood. Donna's mother worked as a restaurant cook, partly to support her four energetic and growing children and partly because she loved to cook. At the end of long days at the restaurant, she brought home magazines that featured pictures of food from all over the world. An inquisitive and confident seven-year-old, Donna didn't see why she couldn't make those foods herself! Of course, it wasn't long before that was exactly what she was doing.

While I spent my days in the clinical laboratory at Michigan looking for ways to improve heart health and defeat heart disease, Donna turned to a laboratory of a different nature: her kitchen. Donna began creating the kinds of meals that spread rumors, and before long students and residents at the university medical school and hospital regularly stopped by my office hoping for an invitation to sit at our dining table. Donna's artistic and delicious meal creations became a living testament to the truth that food that is good for you can also be good to eat! Donna began compiling recipes and menus for meals low in cholesterol, low in fat, and low in sodium.

When I came to Howard University in Washington, D.C., as director of Hypertension/Preventive Cardiology and the Cardiac Intensive Care Unit and subsequently director of the General Clinical Research Center, I wanted to target academic focus on the relationship between obesity and heart disease. Little was being done at the time to study this important connection and Donna and I both believed it was important, actually, *vital*, to do more. Funded by a National Institutes of Health Preventive Cardiology Academic Award (PCAA), the first Obesity Study started. A second PCAA obesity project followed the first, and the third PCAA obesity program became the large-scale Obesity Study from which much of Menu for Life, the concept, evolved. On the clinical end, there were various factors to consider as risks for heart disease. High blood pressure, high blood cholesterol, and diabetes led the list. Doctors also had started noticing that obesity often was present with these health conditions, and that the health problems became worse with obesity. Like other researchers, Donna and I began to suspect that obesity enhanced other health problems and also was itself a health problem. This became part of the hypothesis for the third PCAA obesity program.

The Obesity Study at Howard University's General Clinical Research Center structured a weight loss approach that integrated healthy eating habits with regular exercise, and designed objective tests and measurements to document the results. Donna's catering company, LoChol Gourmet, provided low-fat, low-cholesterol, low-sodium catered meals for participants in the Obesity Study. Donna had one final criterion for the food: it had to taste good. She talked with study participants to learn their favorite foods, and then crafted recipes that presented those foods in healthier ways. Study participants loved them! Donna held cooking workshops to show people how to fix the recipes themselves.

Although we are publishing the results of the study in professional journals to document the evidence linking obesity, health problems, and heart disease, we also felt the strong desire to take our lifetime of knowledge and investigation and create a Menu for Life guide for the people. In *Menu for Life*, we share with you the insights of our experience. As you read, we hope you make this your *personal* Menu for Life. We hope Menu for Life becomes the same kind of catalyst for change in your life that the Obesity Study was for those who participated in it. The outcomes, good or bad, of all ideas both start with and consist of more than one step, one link. When you can envision that first step, you can take it. And the next. And the next. Our Menu for Life now spans the experience of decades, the talents of many people along the way, and the hope for better health for the people whose lives it touches. Where will Menu for Life lead us now? Donna and I are excited to see all the possibilities, and look forward to seeing what will manifest for our Menu for Life in the tomorrows that lay ahead. How far do *you* want *your* Menu for Life to take you?

Acknowledgments

~~~~~~~~

W̶e want to thank everyone who made a contribution to *Menu for Life*. As is the nature of such things, it is not possible for us to name you all but you know who you are and what your contributions have been. Especially, we thank the hundreds of you who participated in the Obesity Study or wanted to participate but could not be accommodated. You are special people!

Dr. Randall thanks these individuals for their unique contributions: Most of all, I thank Donna C. Randall, food artist and chef extraordinaire. Thanks to Park W. Willis, III, M.D., Chief of Cardiology, University of Michigan, a most significant influence from my senior year in medical school through his appointment of me as director of the Cardiac Intensive Care Unit. Thanks also to Andrew Zweifler, M.D., director, Preventive Cardiology Program, University of Michigan, and David Bassett, M.D., and Stevo Julius, M.D., whose teachings continue to influence me, as well as Professor J. K. Alexander, M.D., Baylor College of Medicine, who excited my interest in the cardiovascular pathophysiology of obesity. Thanks to Elaine Stone, M.D., NIH project director for the Preventive Cardiology Academic Award that launched my formal studies of obesity and heart disease. Acknowledgment to Howard University, and appreciation for the staff at the General Clinical Research Center (GCRC) for their dedication and commitment to the Obesity Project, and to Betty M. Deen for her continual contributions. A warm thanks to my parents for the encouragement and unrelenting support they extended to the endeavors of all of their children, especially mine.

Donna Randall gives special thanks to these individuals: I thank Dr. Randall for his belief that preventive medicine offers a better solution to obesity than medication, and extend heartfelt gratitude for the confidence and belief he expressed in my ability to produce meals that would keep the interest of the Obesity Study participants. Thanks to the staff of LoChol Gourmet for their dedication to producing desirable, enticing meals. Special thanks and love to my mother, Dorothy Rideout, and my daughter Cydnee Randall, for the large helping hand they gave to LoChol. Gratitude goes as well to the local newspapers, *The New York Times*, and *Ebony Magazine*, for giving us such wonderful public exposure.

Together, Dr. Randall and Donna Randall both give special thanks to our editor at Broadway Books, Patricia Medved, for her commitment to this book and the importance of its message. Trish's insight into the significance of the Obesity Study led her to place us and the undertaking of writing this book in the capable hands of Lee Ann Chearney at Amaranth, to whom we extend our deepest appreciation and whose vision and talent shaped our experiences into this book; to Deborah S. Romaine, who helped us in putting our voices, theory, and practice on these pages; and to the rest of the Amaranth team for their professionalism and expertise: recipe consultant Eve Adamson, Linda Horning, RD, copyeditor Candace Levy, proofreader Cathy Jewell, and editorial assistants Thomas Kwiczola, Laura Walter, and Katherine Gleason. Thank you to the staff at Broadway including publisher, Gerry Howard, publicist Erin Curtin, publicity director Suzanne Hertz, managing editor Rebecca Holland, editor Frances Jones, assistant Beth Datlowe, and marketing director Catherine Pollock. Finally, we give warm thanks to the six people who participated in the Obesity Study and courageously agreed to share their stories, struggles, and successes with you: Alquietta Brown, Howard Copeland, Stephanie Dove, Marie Primas-Bradshaw, Clarence White, and Cedric Williams.

Part One

~~~~~

More to Love?

1

~~~~~~~~~~

Americans,
African Americans,
and Obesity

We're going to talk to you about what you already know, about what you know better than any book, doctor, nutritionist, husband, wife, child, friend, or minister could tell you—whether you admit it to yourself or not.

Why listen to us? Because we've been there and we understand the frustration and distress you are feeling in your mind and in your body. We want to support and help you. So many things play on your mind when you get to that weight that is beyond where you ever thought you'd be. Well, you can hold on to an image of that thin thing you grew up with, but it would be ideal if you could lose enough weight so that you feel good about who you are—inside and out. We're talking about now. We're talking about today.

We're going to talk to you about what you know when you get up in the morning, already tired and aching. About what you know when you choose your most camouflaging clothes from the closet, and how you feel when you put them on. We're going to talk to you about what you know when you go through your day reaching, bending, and stretching until you get short of breath, until you have to stop and rest, rest just a little while, while people around you keep on going. About what you know when you take the elevator or drive around too long so you can park up close. About what you know when you confront one more time the daily choice to make *another* small compromise to accommodate the slowness, the heaviness. (It's just one *little* thing, right? Doesn't *mean* anything in the long run. . . . You can still do what you've got to do, after all.) We're going to talk to you about what you already know when your doctor says to you, "Your pressure is a little bit high," or "Your sugar is a little bit high," and prescribes pills for you to take or insulin to take, every day, indefinitely.

We're going to talk to you about what you know when you get home exhausted at the end of the day and sink gratefully into your comfortable chair and take solace in the one enjoyment of your life you can indulge in, that fills you up, relaxes your body, and calms your mind. It's there for you: the one source that presents no judgment, only pleasure. The one reward that gives you refuge from all the people, places, and things that cause you stress—food. But when you climb back into bed at night the voice within you kicks up again, your body's aches and pains throb to remind you just how tired you are, how unlike yourself you feel, how difficult it is to move. And after an uncomfortable, fitful night of less than restful sleep, you get up and you have to face it all over again, you have to face what you already know.

Hundreds of people just like you have come to us because of this truth, this truth you already know, but may not be willing to admit. *This heavy person is not the real you.* But for years now, what you've been saying, and really wanting to believe, is just the opposite: "I like being fat." Do you?

For us, the importance of a Menu for Life is more than just a professional calling. We have grappled with the problem of excessive weight gain and the health problems that come with it in our own extended family, which has a history of heart disease on both sides. Donna herself once weighed in at 257 pounds and suffered from high cholesterol.

DONNA RANDALL

"A little over six years ago, I found myself drifting out of the realm of overweight and into that of obesity. The lure of the commercials and advertisements on weight loss brought back the excitement that with the promise of weight loss I would be led back to the exuberant person of my youth. Every new product, pill, piece of exercise equipment I heard about or saw in the media guaranteeing weight loss reminded me of the circus that came to town when I was a child. Caught up in the excitement of the parade and the music of the bandwagon, I wanted to jump on and to be a part of it . . . it was alive.

"Many 'parades' passed by and I tried to jump on the bandwagon each time, only to fail each time. I experienced a terrible letdown with each failure because, in spite of what I had lost, I regained it quickly, plus a little more. Adhering to the prescribed, bland low-cholesterol diet I was given proved to be excessively restrictive. Everything in the 'No' column was what I wanted to eat. The cake was *angel food*. My chocolate cake was gone. I started trying out my own conversions to low-fat, low-sodium, calorie-appropriate and nutrient-dense recipes. These recipes would form the basis of the meals I planned for the obesity study Dr. Randall and I created together. I started putting things back in the 'Yes' column.

"Do I still struggle with my weight? Yes, I do. I will always need to watch my cholesterol and stay vigilant. My family has a history of heart disease; I've had one near heart attack episode myself. My insurance policy is in the form of this book you hold right now in your hands; not just a cookbook, a nutrition or health primer, or an exercise routine, the program Dr. Randall and I co-created, that we present to you here, is truly my—and your—Menu for Life."

DR. RANDALL

"When you get to a certain weight, you develop health problems. You develop high blood pressure. You develop diabetes. It's hard for you to breathe, and your joints hurt and break down. You develop a big heart, because your heart is pumping for two peoples' weight. If you walk around all day with what amounts to two of you and you do this for 10 to 15 years, it will take its toll on your body. Some people say to me, 'How much do I need to lose?' I say, 'You need to lose one half of yourself.' And we laugh about it. But, seriously, your heart would have to work only half as hard if you lost half your weight. The pressure on your joints would lift if you didn't weigh one-and-a-half or two times what you ought to weigh. There's comfort when you lose the weight."

In this book, we're going to speak to that place deep within you, the place that wants to listen and see the truth: the very essence of you, of who you are, your very soul. We *know* you don't want to be heavy. You don't *like* being heavy, no matter what you may say to others in public, or even to yourself in private. But what can you *do* about it? The weight keeps going up—10 pounds, another 10, and then 10 more. You focus, you work hard, and you lose the weight on a diet, and then gain back more. Diets don't work; nothing works. No matter what you do, the pounds keep adding up until you're off the scale. It gets to the point where you don't even want to *know* how many pounds. The years and the pounds add up to an uncomfortable, unrecognizable sum. You stop getting on the scale. You stop looking in the mirror. You stop looking into your own heart.

You wonder if you will ever feel good in your body again. You tell your-self that this is just the way it is—that you have to resign yourself to the weight, find ways to work around it, accept it. Because you feel you have no other choice, because you see no doable solution to this problem, you give in to your weight. You think you have to give in, in order to be able to live with yourself every day.

We're here to tell you that you *can* lose the weight if you want to, keep it off, and live and feel better. Together, we've worked with many people just like you and achieved the results you are longing for, the ones you are convinced right now may never happen for you—positive, healthful results that last when you commit yourself to making it happen, one day at a time, one pound at a time, every day. *"But I've been told this before,"* you say. *"I've tried this before, and it either didn't work, or it didn't last."*

When you see commercials or advertisements for quick weight-loss programs and fad diets and they say at the bottom in fine print, right after the miraculous "success" story, "results not typical." You read those ads, look at their pictures, and tell yourself, "They are setting me up to fail." And you are right about that. Quick weight-loss programs admit the truth right in their own ads: they don't work for most people, and even when they do, the results are not sustained. The day comes when you flip through a magazine and find an ad for a fad diet that is so enticing, so believable, that you jump right back on the roller coaster. And the high is so exhilarating while you are dropping pounds! But then there's the inevitable low when the diet is over and the pounds come back, and then some. Sometimes the pounds come back even more quickly than you lost them. Please know you are not alone. Excessive weight gain is reaching epidemic proportions in America. Americans spend $33 billion a year for products and services to help them lose weight. Yet about a third of peo-ple regain weight lost through diets and special programs within six months; 90 percent gain back their lost weight and add on more within three years.

So, what do you *do?* We've spent our lives figuring this out. Donna Ran-dall and I are partners; the synergies of health and life have shaped and defined our partnership and our goals. Our individual strengths, our weak-nesses, our family, our personal experiences—alone and together—our talents, and our professional training, Donna's as a chef and nutrition expert and my own as a physician, an internist and cardiologist, have led us down a path of mutual investigation. We've searched—just as you are searching now—using our skills to find the recipe, the right ingredients, and method that yield a flavorful, healthful, and satisfying Menu for Life. What are we going to tell you about losing weight that you *don't* already know? We're going to tell you that there *are* methods that work and things you can do to help yourself in a lasting way.

But to begin your journey through our Menu for Life program, you must take one very important step. You must say, *"I can."* Repeat it, *"I can,"* every morning and every night like a prayer. Believe in yourself. Turn your negatives into positives. *"I can lose the weight. I can be whomever I choose to be."* Without this first step, there can be no others. If there is any magic to losing weight, it lives in the part of you that knows who you are and what you want for your life. When you know who you are and what you want to achieve, you can act on your goals with confidence.

What we're talking about is more than "positive thinking." You may work on thinking happy thoughts every day, and that's nice! But happy thoughts by themselves won't take off even one pound. And happy thoughts can't take away the aches and strain on your heart, the frustration, the anger of accepting a way of life that does not make you happy. Who wants to be the fat, happy positive thinker? So we're not talking about a smile to mask your pain. What we're talking about is honest, goal-oriented thinking, taking a look at the way things are in your life and believing that you can change them if you want to. *If you can see it, you can be it.* You can become in real life what you see in your mind's eye. Close your eyes and envision yourself living a life that truly makes you happy. How do you look? How do you feel? Where are you? Who are you with? What are you doing? What you envision may have to do with losing weight, or the weight loss may only be one part of what you see.

You don't just wake up one morning and discover that you weigh twice what you weighed the day before! It might seem that way, but weight gain is a process that takes place over time. A pound a month seems harmless, but it becomes 12 pounds in a year, that 12 pounds becomes 60 pounds in five years, 120 pounds in ten years. Slowly and steadily, excess body fat builds. The heaviness you carry is your unintentional creation, built over time. In the same way, to be permanent, weight loss must also take place over time. It has taken you time to gain the weight, to carry the weight; it will take time to let it go. And change is not always easy. We become accustomed to our habits. Even if we are uncomfortable living in them, we reinforce them year after year. Other people expect us to look and act in certain ways, and we expect the same from ourselves. We are creatures of habit.

But there are compelling reasons to change. You know it; we know it. And we say, *"You can."* You can decide to lose weight, and do it. It is a process of *living*, not of failure or success, or of losing some set number of pounds, or of what the other people in your life have to say that may deter you or set you back. It is a process of creating the person—inside and out—that you want to be, that feels comfortable and is healthy for *you*.

WEIGHT GAIN KNOWS NO RACE OR ETHNICITY

We created the Menu for Life program with our African-American community in mind, but, in truth, our program for reversing excessive weight gain can be used by *anyone*, as the physiological process of weight gain and weight loss knows no ethnicity, race, culture, country, or religion. Some researchers may try to argue otherwise, but we can find no compelling or definitive evidence to support the theory that weight gain is inherently a matter of ethnicity. Weight gain is weight gain, for everyone, period.

Carrying too much weight is not a black problem, a white problem, or a Hispanic problem; carrying too much weight is a *human* problem, an *American* problem. Americans weigh more with each passing year. Six in ten Americans are overweight, and one in four qualifies for what doctors term "clinically obese," according to figures released by the U.S. Centers for Disease Control and Prevention (CDC). This means that more than half of all Americans—more than 100 *million* people—weigh too much. Even more disturbing, the frequency of obesity in the United States rose 30 percent in the decade between 1980 and 1990 alone and shows no signs of letting up. We are gaining weight by the minute and getting fatter every day. Obesity is not just our problem; it is our family's problem, our children's problem. Since 1980, adolescents are three times more likely to be overweight; in 1999 13 percent of children and adolescents fit the doctor's clinical definition of obese. We are passing our weight problem along to our children in the example we are setting with our own lives.

So, we are not talking about a few individuals putting on a few pounds here and there, easily gained in a weekend's indulgence and lost in a week's efforts of self-discipline. We are talking about a national trend that does not discriminate, a trend toward obvious and excessive weight gain in ourselves and in our children that occurs steadily over months, years, and decades in households all over the United States, from the cities to the plains—north, south, east, and west. We are talking about a generation of Americans who eat more and move less than any generation in our nation's history. In a telephone survey conducted in 2000 and reported in the *Journal of the American Medical Association,* 27 percent of people responding told researchers they "did not engage in any physical activity," and 28 percent described themselves to researchers as "not regularly active." But we know, once again, that we are not telling you anything that you don't already know and see all around you. You don't need statistics like these for you to know that overweight people are everywhere, moving less with every pound they gain.

How Many Pounds Really *Are* Too Many?

Some of us, though, are tempted to take comfort in belonging to the overweight majority, and this, sadly, is a point of view too often held by black people. After all, how can extra pounds be *that* bad when so many people seem to be doing just fine? Isn't it better and healthier to have a few extra pounds of stored energy on our bodies than to walk around without any energy reserves? Food, after all, is nourishment, and logic would seem to tell us that eating more food must certainly be better than eating less food.

However, thanks to advances in technology as well as people's increased longevity, doctors and nutritionists have learned much in the past 20 years or so about how what we eat influences our health for better or worse. Today, scientists can tell you how your body uses each bite of food you swallow—how your body breaks that food into chemical substances, where those substances go, and how they help or harm your overall health. All of this new information refutes cultural assumptions throughout history that an ever bigger body is a sign of increased health and well-being. In future chapters we're going to talk to you about the specifics of the physiological process of excessive weight gain and just how and why it is *not* good for your body.

When you gain too much weight, it is difficult to see all the damage that is taking place *inside* your body. From the *outside*, it can seem to appear that your too-heavy body may be equally as healthy as the not-so-heavy body of the person waiting behind you in the grocery store check-out line. In your mind's eye, take a moment to observe that other person you imagine. Does she breathe more easily than you do? Can she reach the items on the bottom of the cart without a struggle? Does she move quickly to catch the oranges that escape from their bag and start to roll along the counter? Can she bend effortlessly to pick up that bag of white flour corn chips her toddler tosses onto the linoleum floor? (We hope that the toddler you conjure with your mind's eye hasn't been eating those chips in the grocery store. No child should eat food while rolling or walking through the grocery aisles!) If the answer to all of these questions is yes, then you might want to consider what these signs mean.

We're not saying you need to be able to leap over the aisle displays and do a four-second dash Jackie Joyner-Kersee style down the frozen food lane to consider yourself in shape. (Though if you want to imagine yourself doing that, enjoy the run! Remember, seeing something in your mind's eye is the first step toward making it real.) And we're not saying everyone needs to become thin, whatever "thin" means to you. What we are saying is that a real-world trip to the grocery store should not leave you feeling like you earned enough points to win a heptathlon.

In your mind's eye when you see people who are too thin, are a healthy weight, are a few pounds overweight, a bit more than a few pounds overweight, or definitely more than overweight, seriously overweight, extremely overweight, what do they look like, to *you*? Remember, nearly *half* of the people you see every day are overweight to some degree. Are you sure you can identify what a person of healthy weight looks like? Forget about the reed thin actress's or buffed-up actor's impossible ideal on the movie screen—who knows if that's real or computer-enhanced? We mean: do you know what an everyday person on the street of healthy weight looks like? How about your *own* weight? Having too much weight, some people rationalize, does not mean they could be obese, just a "plus" size.

When you look at the people around you, you will notice that in addition to being of all sizes, they are of all shapes. No two bodies are the same. Some bodies are solid and squared, while others are rounded and soft. To a great extent, you must live in the body type you have been given in this life. If you are short, for example, you will always be short; pound for pound, you may look heavier than people who weigh the same as you but are taller.

In our experience, many people have a mistaken idea about how much weight is too much—and they also fail to recognize when that weight starts causing them health problems. Doctors, when they give you a physical examination, will take your height and weight, and they will use these figures as objective indicators to determine where your weight is on a scale of healthy weight to unhealthy weight. From your height and weight, doctors calculate a number called the Body Mass Index (BMI). BMI is a mathematical formula that converts height and weight figures into a scale of values rated according to potential health risk. (We'll help you calculate your BMI in Chapter 4.) Here is how health professionals view the relationship between weight, BMI, and health:

- UNDERWEIGHT *BMI under 18.5*
  The range of weight, for your height, at which your body is likely receiving inadequate nutrition. Though the health risks of underweight differ from those of overweight or obesity, they can be equally dangerous.
- HEALTHY WEIGHT *BMI of 18.5 to 24.9*
  The range of weight, for your height, at which there is no increase in your risk for health problems or for diseases where there is a known correlation to body weight.
- OVERWEIGHT *BMI of 25 to 29.9*
  The range of weight, for your height, at which your weight begins to affect body functions such as insulin sensitivity (important to people with diabetes). At this weight range excess body fat is generally present but might not be that obvious, and clothing sizes are still "average." It is possible—and common—for people to be overweight and healthy. For example, you might weigh more than a height/weight chart of healthy weight values recommends if you are involved in strenuous athletic activities that increase your muscle mass (muscle weighs more than fat). However, for most people this classification is where problems may begin to start.
- MODERATELY OBESE *BMI of 30 to 34.9*
  The range of weight, for your height, at which your risk for certain health problems increases. Excess body fat appears obvious, and there is enough of an increase in body mass to affect functions such as blood

pressure. You are likely to shop for at least some of your clothing in "plus" or "big man" sizes.

- SERIOUSLY OBESE *BMI of 35 to 39.9*

  The range of weight, for your height, at which you face significant risk for certain health problems. You are obese if your percentage of body fat is 20 percent or more than that of people of healthy weight for your height. At this weight range, all of your clothing is "plus" or "big man" sized.

- EXTREMELY OBESE *BMI of 40 and higher*

  The range of weight, for your height, that places you at extreme risk for multiple health problems. This classification generally identifies people who weigh 100 pounds or more than the healthy weight value for their height, and are more likely than not to have at least one obesity-related health problem. At this weight range, it is difficult to find clothing that fits you.

Weight for Height Ranges

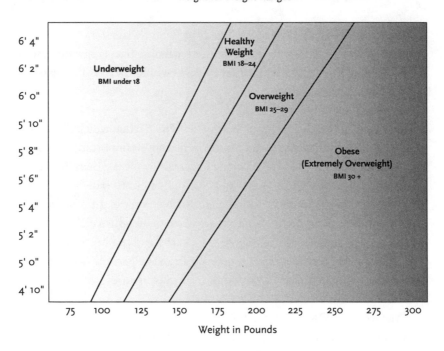

Where Does Your Weight Fall in This Graph?

EXTRA WEIGHT DOESN'T HELP—IT HURTS!

Even with objective evidence and a doctor's advice that weight loss is needed to improve their health, we've seen people cling to the idea that their weight is okay, even desirable. But why say, *I can*, and start losing weight if you believe that extra weight is helping you instead of hurting you? When Donna gives cooking demonstrations, she often hears people try to justify eating too much by saying their boyfriends want them to appear more curvaceous or their girlfriends like them big and strong—it's more feminine or more masculine to have that extra weight. "*More to love,*" they tell her. Maybe you believe this too. We hear it all the time. In answer, Donna likes to refer to that old saying, the one a lot of women grew up with in the 1950s, "*The only way to a man's heart is through his stomach.*" Donna will tell you, "You feed your husband what you are going to eat yourself. But what you don't understand is that in pleasing your man's stomach—and your own stomach too—you are damaging his heart as well as your own. What good is gaining your true love's heart with food, if that food is only going to put that person's precious health in jeopardy?"

Today, food—an often endless choice of food—is seldom more than minutes away. If you don't feel like fixing something from your kitchen, it's likely just a short drive to a fast-food restaurant where you can "super-size" your selection to get even more food for your money. And oftentimes, we don't eat because we are hungry or because we need to eat to ensure our physical survival. We don't eat to make ourselves healthier or more attractive. We eat because we can; we eat because the food is there. If anything, we eat to ensure our *emotional* survival; to reduce stress because we feel good in that moment while we are eating. When we eat, we are able to satisfy ourselves, to feel substantial. Most times though, we probably don't think too much about the food we put in our mouths. We eat what we like. We eat what is easy or convenient or simply at hand. But the body weight we pack on because we eat too much—because we just cannot resist that deep-fried catfish fillet—rather than carrying us through tough times or turning our troubles into joys just makes us fat. Weight causes more problems than it will ever solve.

Too much weight, excessive weight, is not healthy. A few pounds, in and of themselves, may not be a problem, but sustained, uninterrupted weight gain combined with a very low level of physical activity leads to serious health problems. We want you to learn how to stop gaining and how to keep the weight off once you do start losing. Donna and I both believe strongly that a positive, lasting synergy for health and for life, our mutual Menu for Life—Donna's, mine, and yours—must start here, in this moment of realization that too much weight, and the physical slowness that accompanies it, is not good. Our hope is that this message reaches your soul before you or someone you love experience a catastrophic health problem from which you may, or may not, be able to recover. Unless you commit to saying *I can*, unless you believe in yourself and believe you *can* —and *should*—lose the weight, you won't. You will simply continue to hide from the truth. And that's no recipe for living.

As a cardiologist, I treat many patients who are people I see for the first time when they are admitted to the intensive care unit or the coronary care unit, fighting for their lives. I give them all that medical technology can offer. For those who survive, I know that the experience is a wake-up call to a sobering reality: if they are too heavy, their weight is killing them. Former Surgeon General Dr. David Satcher released a report in 2001 documenting that 300,000 Americans die every year from diseases, such as heart disease and several types of cancer, that have obesity as a risk factor; compare that to 400,000 who die as a consequence of smoking. "Overweight and obesity may soon cause as much preventable disease and death as cigarette smoking," Dr. Satcher warns. He is right. Today, we are experiencing an epidemic of obesity. But we are only just beginning to understand the extent to which, pound for pound, we are laying the foundation for a second epidemic, the consequences of obesity.

We know that mortality goes up when weight goes up. If your weight is one-and-a-half times as much as it should be, your odds of dying double. How can that be, you ask. Don't we *all* have 100 percent chance of dying at any given time? After all, occasionally people do get hit by lightning or buses! That's true. We're talking odds, though, not certainty. If you go to a horse race, it is reasonably certain that all the horses will cross the finish line. The statistical odds that each horse will finish first, second, third, and so on, however, are something else entirely. We are all certain to cross life's finish line, but when? *If your weight is one-and-a-half times as much as it should be, your odds of dying double.* If you weigh 210 pounds and you are standing next to a person of the same height and gender who weighs 140 pounds, you are twice as likely to cross the finish line of life before the other person. And, statistically, as your weight continues to increase, your odds of dying increase, literally, at an exponential rate. These are not desirable odds if long life is among your personal objectives. If "eat, drink, and be merry while the sun shines" means to you that you may as well pack on the pounds because we're all going to die someday anyway and what difference does it make, your day may come sooner than you think.

If you look at two groups of people, one group that is of healthy weight and one that is overweight, people in each group will have diabetes, high blood pressure, kidney disease, and heart disease. But the group that is overweight will have four to six times as many health problems—or more—than the group that is of healthy weight. Obesity, having a BMI of 30 or greater, is what we in the health profession call an "independent risk factor." Other factors aside, your risk for health problems and even early death rises correspondingly with your weight.

CREATING A MENU FOR LIFE PROGRAM FOR AFRICAN AMERICANS

Earlier in this chapter we told you that we do not believe that weight gain or loss has anything to do with ethnicity or race. However, the relationship between obesity and some diseases and conditions that are more prevalent in African Americans than in the general population, such as high blood pressure, heart disease, high cholesterol, and diabetes, conspires to cause special problems for black people. This is especially true for black women, who, among all Americans, have the highest incidence of excessive weight gain. Sixty-six percent of black women are overweight. One in ten black women is extremely overweight, over 100 pounds more than the healthy weight for their height. At least 60 percent of all African Americans are overweight by age 60. For black men, the relationship of kidney disease to high blood pressure and obesity is a subject of ongoing study. Between the ages of 25 and 44, African Americans, especially black men, are on dialysis an alarming 18 to 20 times more than anyone else. If all this scares you, Donna and I think that is an appropriate and healthy response. But over the years, Donna and I came to believe that many of these life-and-death crises African Americans face because of obesity could be prevented.

In 15 years of daily rounds as the director of the Cardiac Intensive Care Unit at the University of Michigan and at Howard University Hospital, I noted that patients with no appreciable risk factors for heart disease rarely have heart attacks or evidence of atherosclerosis, the accumulation of fatty substances and cellular debris that cling to the walls of the arteries and that eventually restrict the flow of blood to the heart. People who show three or more risk factors, who participate in risky behaviors for heart disease, are more likely to experience coronary artery disease (CAD)—the number one cause of cardiovascular deaths in the United States. Risk factors for heart disease include smoking, eating fatty foods, not exercising, gaining too much weight, and/or a family history of heart disease. A family history of heart disease can be defined as a risk factor people can't control, but can only inherit, or it also can mean acquiring the undesired behaviors that put people at greater risk. Taking a look at this pattern of health and illness, Donna and I began to believe, as did other researchers, that lifestyle factors could significantly affect cardiovascular health.

Then we took it one step further. Could reversing or preventing excessive weight gain—obesity—*alone* result in reversing or preventing cardiovascular and other disease conditions? If so, the health benefits for African Americans, in particular, would be dramatic and lasting. All people had to do to lower their risks for heart attacks, we postulated, would be to improve nutrition, eat less food, and increase their activity, enough to bring about *even a modest weight loss.* Along with weight loss, receiving treatment under a doctor's care could reduce or eliminate, if possible, other damaging health conditions, such as high blood pressure, high cholesterol, or diabetes.

Donna and I envisioned a structured program to help African Americans lose weight to improve their health situations. We would monitor and study the physiological, nutritional, and anecdotal data the program generated to evaluate, refine, and enhance a synergistic prescription for health and well-being. The Obesity Study, conducted at Howard University's General Clinical Research Center (GCRC), was initiated during a five-year National Institutes of Health (NIH) preventive cardiology academic award to make medical students aware of and to teach them about methods and techniques to prevent cardiovascular disease. Together through the Obesity Study, the GCRC and staff, Donna and I have helped over 300 people make the lifestyle changes necessary to lose weight and keep it off using our Menu for Life.

In groups of about 50 people at a time, study participants agreed to go through a six-month program that combined three supplied nutritious meals a day, prepared by Donna within an 1,800 to 2,000 calorie daily target, with cooking seminars and food demonstrations, health seminars and monitoring, and 45 minutes of walking on a treadmill, at a minimum, three times each week. In this book, we're going to lay out this weight-loss, health-enhancing program for you. This is a Menu for Life that allows you to eat with joy and live with vitality.

Now, Donna, she is not just a cook; I call her a *food artist*, because she goes into the kitchen with the same creativity and intelligence of a painter or a musician. She enjoys preparing good food that people will like that also meets all the health requirements. "For people to stay in the Menu for Life program," Donna says, "they have to like the food and want to eat it." Donna set about creating a healthy, low-fat, low-sodium, calorie-appropriate, nutrient-dense meal plan that people participating in the study could eat without giving up the tastes and flavors they loved. In this book, Donna will tell you what you need to know about nutrition and health. She'll tell you how to shop, cook, and eat healthfully; give you recipes that are delicious, and make sure you are getting the right nutrients to meet the daily requirements that will promote health; and help you plan meals that nourish you and fill you up. Believe me, forget about being disappointed by the food; Donna's recipes will be more than enough to satisfy. "I tell people, *you can have your chocolate cake and eat it too* and still lose weight," Donna says. "You *can*. Literally."

Some people who participated with us in the Menu for Life program lost over 100 pounds, while others lost 30 to 40 pounds. But all of them left the study pleased with the improvements they felt in their health and saw in their appearance and hopeful that they could continue their new eating and exercise habits on their own to meet the goals they had established for themselves. Many have been successful; some have continued to struggle. Their stories are real and inspirational, and these six people have agreed to share their experiences with you throughout the pages of this book:

- Cedric Williams weighed over 350 pounds when he suffered a debilitating stroke at age 38. Cedric lost 150 pounds in 10 months, and has kept the weight off for three years and counting. His diabetes and his high blood pressure are under control without medication. "The hardest part is getting started," Cedric says. "But this is not a contest, it is a lifetime commitment."
- Stephanie Dove had a cardiac event at age 44, after which her doctor told her that if she didn't lose weight she would die. She went from 220

pounds to 165 pounds in six months, but then gained back 20 pounds in the eight months after completing the program, although she is determined to lose it again and keep it off. "It's about living long enough to see my child grow up," says Stephanie.

• Clarence White, a retired Army man, found himself at age 63 with 230 pounds on his six-foot frame. Clarence took medications for everything from high blood pressure to asthma, gout, and high cholesterol. With a family history of adult onset diabetes, Clarence wanted to minimize his experience of, and risk for, health problems. He lost 35 pounds, now weighs in at about 195, and takes only two medications. "All that you can do, it will only help. What I acquired in the program will take me through the rest of my life."

• Marie Primas-Bradshaw entered the weight-reduction program because she wanted to do something good for herself. She lost 40 pounds in six months and hopes to lose another 35 pounds to get to her ideal weight. "This is a journey," says Marie. "You're going to feel you have some tough road ahead. But it's a sense of command, not control. And it's exciting, in a way that stays and grows."

• Howard Copeland tried diet after diet to shed the pounds that had begun to cause health problems, and then he entered the weight-reduction program at the recommendation of a friend who was already in it. He lost 30 pounds in four months and plans to lose another 15 pounds so he can stop taking medication for his blood pressure. "I'm doing this just for me," Howard says. "I'm very happy with how I look and feel."

• Alquietta Brown, a nurse at Howard University Hospital on the unit adjacent to Dr. Randall's, entered the program when she found out she had diabetes and needed to take insulin. At 35, Alquietta weighed over 200 pounds, but lost just over 60 pounds in a two-year period. For the most part, she's been able to keep the weight off. By the time she left the study, Alquietta's blood sugar was normal. "I don't need to take oral medications or insulin and I'm thrilled, because I didn't want to do that."

Over the years, Donna and I learned so much, not only from the health and nutritional information we gathered and examined—and that we're going to share with you in this book—but also from those unique and special individuals, every one of the 300 who passed through our lives, who allowed us to help them create a synergy of health and well-being, by moving more, making smarter food choices, and watching their health, so they could lose weight in order to feel better. And, we hope they took what they learned from us home to their families, to share with them the benefit of longer, happier, healthier lives.

YOUR MENU FOR LIFE: LOOKING FROM THE INSIDE OUT

This you already know: you don't go on diets or start weight-loss programs because you are happy with how you look and feel. And you are not reading this book because you are happy with how you look and feel. We know that when you are heavy and you want to lose weight, only losing weight will make you happy. You do it one pound at a time. You lose one pound, and that is great. You lose 10 pounds, and that is great too. You lose what you *want* to lose. You do it by changing your lifestyle. You eat healthfully, and you become more active. You focus on the improvements in your health, and over time, one day at a time, everything else falls into place. If you have a week every now and then where you gain a pound, well, that is going to happen. If you have a health setback, you can get the medical attention you need and set about making the changes that will deal with that too. Forget about having to comply with some idea of success or failure—some number of pounds you need to lose or some set time frame in which you feel you need to lose them. Forget about achieving any goal that comes anywhere but from inside *you*. Remember that weight loss is not an "outside in" proposition. It is an "inside out" process. It takes time. Be patient, be persistent, be curious, and be tenacious. Be *yourself*. Every day, repeat like a prayer, *"I can."*

Donna says, "Each of us must navigate the intricate maze of life. And only *you* know how to be the best at being *you*. I cannot tell you who you are. What I *can* tell you is this: who and what you are starts with what you accept from *yourself*. If you find you are dissatisfied with your state of being, change it. Not because someone told you to change, but because you want to. Anything else will end in frustration.

"We want to know how you are doing and what we can do to help you do this better, your personal process of weight loss and change from the inside out. Keep reading, and we will go with you. We will help you create the menu for *your* life. It is an honor and a privilege—an enrichment to the synergy of our lives, Dr. Randall's and mine—to get to know you."

2

~~~~~~~~~

Why We Overeat

Look around you. What do you see? Big. Everything is big. We buy big, eat big, live big. *Bigger is better*. Get a lot for your money, and all that goes with it. Sometimes extra—two for one. We shop in "big box" superstores and warehouse stores, walk down wide aisles, and buy in bulk. The economy package gives us more of whatever product it is we want to have, more of it for less money. And we enjoy getting more for our hard-earned dollars. We *search* for ways to get more productivity out of those dollars. We load up our purchases in the trunks of our cars and ride home. And if we are running behind (because there is never enough time and far too much to do), we rush to the drive-through to pick up a bucket or box of something for the family dinner and call it a day.

Today, *bigger is better* is the American way of life. The message is taking hold and too many of us believe it is true. As a result, we consume more and more. We are bigger; our kids are bigger. The bigger is better message is so pervasive that it is harder and harder in our country—no matter what race, ethnicity, gender, or age you are—to get away from it. Look around you. Bigger is better is everywhere. We *demand* more for less, and we are happy when we get it.

But when you eat more and move less, like most of us do these days, your body can only get so big before something has to give. After a certain point, it is harder and harder to convince yourself that a bigger body is better. You feel it in your bones: you are unhappy with how big your body is and the problems that your weight causes for you. Sometimes you just keep eating anyway. More times, though, this is when you decide to go on a diet. And because you have gone through the cycle of weight loss and weight gain before in your life, it is easy to believe that you can just continue this way.

When bigger becomes uncomfortable, you know you can always decide to scale back. Even if you keep eating past that point of realization and discomfort and gain a few *more* unwanted pounds. You can diet. You can start exercising. After all, *you* are in control of your weight, right? Weight loss and weight gain might well be a cycle that repeats itself over two or three decades of your life. If you get a little bit bigger on each "up" part of the cycle, the "down" part of the cycle likely stays a little higher on each round too. So even if you lose more weight this time than you did on the last round, your weight doesn't get as low.

You keep getting bigger. You lose 20 pounds, and six months or a year later those 20 pounds are back with another two to five pounds added on. You give up for a while, and then you find yourself searching desperately for a solution. You know a solution *must* be out there; it *has* to be! The situation requires action. Because your weight problem just keeps getting bigger, extreme solutions begin to seem the only way out. They lure you with their promises: fad diets that starve your body and provide unbalanced, inadequate nutrition; exercise that is too harsh for your heavy body to bear. The solutions are too stressful, too much to take. So you stop. And the cycle of weight gain starts again.

DONNA RANDALL

"Okay, what are you talking about when you are talking about diet? What is it with our obsession with this word? According to the dictionary, everything we eat is a diet. So you're on a diet. Every day. Case closed. We have to stop talking about a diet as if it is something special, something we impose upon ourselves that shapes and sculpts us from the outside in as if by magic— and all you need to do is follow it. The real question is, how do you survive on a day-to-day basis? What *choices* are you making? What's going on *inside*?

"Menu for Life is not a fad diet; it is choosing healthful food that you enjoy eating, combined with joyous movement that you can put your whole body into. We are talking about something you can live with every day, that doesn't hurt you or leave you hungry. And to do it you don't have to adopt intense training programs like tennis stars Serena and Venus Williams and basketball player Kobe Bryant do. But I can guarantee you this, if you believe you can lose the weight and you start on a Menu for Life, you will *feel* like a pro—and you will share a pro's winning focus of attention, of commitment to working toward a goal of healthful excellence. You'll see your Menu for Life take healthy shape from within yourself—both physically and mentally—and only then will you see lasting changes on the outside."

DR. RANDALL: ~~

"When you first start the Menu for Life program, your body's energy is out of balance. You are putting more energy into your body than you are getting out of it. As long as this continues, your weight moves up the scale. The first thing Donna and I need to help you do is not to lose weight, but to *stop gaining*. This is a *major accomplishment*, and it is so achievable. You want to lose weight, and that is good. But first, you must stop gaining it. If you learn to bring your body into a balance where you are not putting on any additional weight and hold that steady state of balance, you lay the groundwork for a healthful approach to weight loss. When you are in healthy balance, you are less likely to fall victim to an unhealthy pattern of yo-yo weight loss and weight gain. You begin to understand how your body works. You feel better, calmer, more centered. You are more active. You make better choices for yourself and for your family."

Seven in ten African-American women are overweight. If you are one of these seven, you weigh at least 10 percent, or 15 to 20 pounds, more than is healthy. But two in five black women weigh so much that they are obese—weighing at least 20 percent more, 25 pounds or greater, than is healthy. Six in ten black men are overweight, and two of those six are obese. When you weigh so much that you are obese, you have health problems. Your weight and your health problems control your life.

Why do we overeat? We overeat because we can, because we are encouraged to do it. We think less than we should about what we are doing to ourselves because our big bodies have become the new normal. We weigh more and are less active today than 20, 30, or 40 years ago. We need to understand what that means. We are living, and we are raising our children, in a different world.

REWIND, FAST FORWARD: HOW TIMES HAVE CHANGED

Fifty years ago, in the 1950s, African Americans listened to Lena Horne's blues ballads, watched the rise of young actor Sidney Poitier in break-through Broadway shows and Hollywood movies, and thrilled at the magic of Jackie Robinson and the Brooklyn Dodgers' Boys of Summer. In the cru-cible of the civil rights movement, future Supreme Court Justice and then-NAACP lawyer, Thurgood Marshall, argued *Brown v. Board of Education of Topeka, Kansas*, while Rosa Parks's act of courage sparked the Mont-gomery bus boycott. From these times, future Nobel Peace Prize–winner Martin Luther King, Jr., emerged as a civil rights leader of worldwide influ-ence, whose nonviolent protests urged that people be judged by the con-tent of their characters.

When African Americans embarked on the civil rights movement, fast food restaurants didn't exist as we know them today. The closest thing to fast food was the automat! Plastic-wrapped, mass-produced packaged foods were a novelty, not a necessity. Not everyone owned a television (forget about computers or cell phones!) or a car. No drive-throughs. Most Amer-icans, African Americans included, ate at home as charter members in the "clean plate" club. Generations of kids learned from adults to eat every-thing on their plates, *all of it*, no matter what or how much or how little of it there was. After dinner, kids went outside to play while parents did whatever chores needed doing around the house, washing and drying dishes by hand and maybe even washing the kitchen floor on their hands and knees. On special evenings, the adults went out to play cards with friends, dance, or listen to jazz. No videos, no big screen TVs, no home entertainment centers.

Back then, doctors didn't know what we know now about the correla-tions between what we eat, how we move, and our health. Researchers suspected but didn't yet have the scientific evidence to support the connection between dietary saturated fat and heart disease. Doctors then believed diabetes to be a disease of sugar and told people who developed diabetes: you can't have sugar anymore. Today, doctors know diabetes is a disease of insulin, either a lack of production or inability to use (insulin resistance), and we tell people with diabetes to maintain balance among the nutrients in the foods they eat and to get regular exercise.

Even 30 years ago, in the 1970s, people didn't eat like we do now, and they didn't live such inactive lives. Cleaning your plate as a kid 30 years ago still meant that you ate a variety of foods someone cooked for you, and even though you had to eat everything on your plate, it was usually a reasonable, or as your mother might have said, a "healthy" amount of food. This seemed a good way to make sure you got enough to eat, for you to understand the value of food, and to get you to eat foods you might otherwise refuse, like green beans or cooked carrots. Maybe you had one or two overweight relatives, and there were perhaps one or two "fat kids" in your class at school, but for the most part the people around you managed to stay at a reasonable weight. Even 20 years ago, in the 1980s, you could buy food in bulk quantities or economy packaging only from wholesale outlets that sold to restaurants, other stores for resale purposes, or to organizations like schools and church kitchens that fed groups of people.

Fast forward to today, and you see a different world. Many things have changed, and for the better. We enjoy the fruits of the civil rights movement when we look around and see African Americans in positions of influence all over our nation. In our time, Sidney Poitier wins an Oscar from Hollywood for Lifetime Achievement and young African-American director Spike Lee makes acclaimed films. Mae Jemison is the first African-American astronaut. Toni Morrison wins the Nobel Prize for Literature. African Americans are CEOs, politicians, physicians, scientists, poets, artists, soldiers, parents, and visionaries. We work to increase our share in the American abundance. Sometimes, yes, bigger is better. Living big can be something grand and beautiful.

But go to your child's school and the classroom is full of overweight children and teenagers. Look around in your neighborhood, at the mall, at church. Living big in America today—for African Americans and *all* Americans—also means gaining pounds and ever bigger bodies. This we must change. On this, we can do better. The amount of food all Americans consider typical is a whole lot more today than it was even 10 years ago in the 1990s, and certainly more than when you were growing up and could seemingly eat "anything" without gaining an ounce.

WEIGHT LOSS AND WEIGHT GAIN ARE BIG BUSINESS

In the 1950s, before fast food and prepared foods took over the market—ostensibly to make our lives easier—Americans spent about $100 million a year on weight-management programs and diet products. Today, in the first decade of the 21st century, we spend *$50 billion a year* in the hope of losing weight! Adjusted for inflation, $100 million in 1950 dollars equals slightly less than three-quarters of $1 billion in 2000 dollars. So, we are spending approximately *50 times as much:* 50 times as much in 50 years. What tangible benefit do Americans get for this $50 billion a year? Not what we expect to get when we put that money out, that's for sure: only *5 in 100* people manage to keep weight off lost through diets and special programs for longer than two years. How can it be that we are *so* willing to spend *so much* of our money on weight-loss products that fail to deliver their promise?

Because we all want to lose weight—because we all want to believe this time will be different—and companies exist to sell us what we want, *over and over again.* When *95 percent* of the people who spend their money on weight-loss programs and products fail to reach or maintain their weight-loss targets, repeat business is strong. You *want to believe* that of the 50 million Americans of every color who are right now, at this very moment, trying to lose weight, you will be among the 5 percent who succeed. If everyone who tried a diet plan or weight loss program actually lost weight and kept it off, there would be no weight loss industry.

Companies thrive on taking what looks to be an overwhelmingly sure bet that you will fail to keep off the weight that you lose. Odds are good too that you *will* return to try a new weight-loss product in the future. Because more often than not, you blame *yourself* for gaining weight back, not the diet or the product. You are perfectly willing and eager to go ahead and try again. Companies win your dollars, all the while knowing full well that your failure to reach your goal of sustainable weight loss ensures their financial success. Take a look at the next weight-loss program brochure you get in the mail and see how much of the pitch is aimed at making you feel comfortable being heavy—makeup tips for women, gut-slimming tips for men, hair-style tips, clothing and accessory tips that "lengthen" and "flatter." Dress it up; bigger is better!

African Americans, especially women, have come to accept heavier bodies. Each time the cycle swings back to putting on a few more pounds, we tell ourselves this is not so bad, that it is healthy and right to love our substantial bodies. After all, Patti LaBelle wears more than a size two and Charles Barkley is the "round mound of rebound." One step forward, two steps back. However, we believe you can do something much more worthy with your energy. And you must believe so too, because you are reading this book, because you are willing to consider a new Menu for Life.

Even as the weight-loss industry beckons, every time you read a magazine, see a billboard, watch television, surf the Internet, or listen to the radio, you encounter advertisements trying to get you to buy food. The US Department of Agriculture (USDA) reports that the food industry spends more than *$12 billion* a year to sell Americans food. This accounts for 16 percent of all advertising, making it the largest advertising segment in the United States after automobile promotions. This $12 billion must be money well spent by advertisers, because we spend more than four times as much a year trying to lose weight.

How can advertisements for food, and food packages (themselves advertising), be *so* seductive? Many researchers, including the US Department of *Energy*, no less, are discovering that the mere sight of food stimulates the brain to release dopamine, a neurotransmitter that carries the message of *pleasure*. You see food, and you want to eat it. Because we need food to survive, it makes sense that our brains do this. What does not make sense is that we are eating more than we need to survive and thrive. Advertising becomes our cultural message to eat, not just when we are hungry, but whenever we want to—because the food is always available. Food seduces our minds and our bodies, and we behave like food addicts.

Because there is no way to keep *overeating* without gaining weight, we enter a cycle of emotional eating where we overindulge and gain, deprive ourselves with diets, overindulge and gain, deprive ourselves with diets. Invariably, we return to the perceived comfort, mental and physical, of food. We return to our old habits of shopping to get more for our money by buying the "value" quantities of food dangled before our eyes and then eating it all. But when there's just you and your kids, or just you by yourself, this is far more food than you need to buy at one time. And it's no bargain if the "value" amount is two, or three, or more times the amount of food that is healthful to eat in a single sitting.

Each year we spend more total dollars for the food we eat. Much of what we pay for is convenience. Manufacturers spend the biggest chunk of their advertising dollars—$7 billion—trying to convince us to buy their brands, mostly of packaged food products. With people working longer hours while raising families, pressed for time and money, manufacturers shrewdly market food kits. Go into the grocery store today and you'll find food kits that put cheese spread in with your nachos, dressing and croutons in with your salad, kits that contain everything you need to *assemble* your pizza, your sandwich, your chicken dinner, whatever it is that you are having. Go ahead; it is *so* easy, *so* tempting. Ready to fix. Microwavable. Everything you need to *help* you in the kitchen, complete from a box or a bag. And the marketing works. Sales of these foods account for an increasingly significant share of your grocery purchases.

You may be getting convenience for your dollar, but are you *really* getting what you *want* to eat? Does this food look or taste all that *good?* Is it fresh? Or is it full of chemicals? Maybe it is just the bag or box that is so appealing. We don't know about you, but we like to choose and prepare our *own* food. Do you *really* need a company to tell you what to put on your sandwich? Besides the boring blandness of eating what's actually *in* that box or bag, processed foods generally have high dietary fat and/or high sodium content combined with low nutritional content. So despite what health or other claims the box or bag might advertise on the front (Trust us, saying on the label that a food is "no fat" is NOT an all-you-can-eat invitation!), or how appetizing the picture on the package looks, or how easy the food seems to fix, most processed foods are far from healthful. You actually get more for your money, in terms of nutritional value, flavor, variety, enjoyment, and health, when you buy fresh foods and ingredients and prepare your family's meals yourself.

But it takes more than just starting to cook again. (And cooking at home is easier than you think!) It means learning *how* to cook in a way that is healthful but still gives you the tastes and flavors you crave. Just as we know now what we didn't know back then about smoking—that it kills—nutrition experts know that our comfort food favorites from childhood—those tastes and flavors many of us can't live without, things like smothered chicken, fried fish, pies, cakes, and cookies—are not the healthiest choices when we prepare them in the traditional high-fat, high-sodium way and eat them all the time and in large portions. Still, that's the way most of us prepare our favorites. When you really want these foods, but you don't want to cook, you can get them "to go" from just about any restaurant or even from the grocery store. Or even easier: pick up the phone and call out—have the food delivered to you.

"I just *loved* my food," says Cedric Williams. "Food was my comfort. I was tired when I came home, and I wanted something to make me feel good. So I'd sit on the couch, watch TV, order take-out food, have it delivered, and pay with my credit card. I didn't even have to get up off the couch, and I could get as much to eat as I wanted."

When Cedric's weight eventually hit more than 350 pounds (he now weighs a much healthier 200 pounds), even sitting on the couch took effort. Friends and family joked that he wouldn't need to stuff his shirt with a pillow when he played Santa during the holidays. And then, at age 38, Cedric had a stroke. "I'd been heavy all my adult life. People called me the Big Guy, I really didn't care. My doctors told me for years about all my health problems, told me that I had to lose weight, *but I thought I felt good,*" he says. "I loved to eat, thought I was breaking new ground. I got on an airplane one time and they had to get me a seat belt extender and other people around me were embarrassed. But I thought it was funny. Really, I was dying and I didn't know it. I was eating myself to death."

We're looking for food that's fast, whether we have it delivered, take it home, or eat at a restaurant. The fast food industry has grown by 60 percent since 1991 and shows no signs of slowing, spending $3 billion a year in advertising. In 1980, fast food advertising accounted for about 5 percent of food advertising expenses; by 1997 it accounted for 28 percent. Never mind that *one* typical fast food "value" meal provides as many calories as you should consume in an entire day. Today Americans spend nearly the same amount of money on fast food purchases ($110 billion a year) as we do for the health care services that treat problems related to obesity (over $117 billion a year). And Americans have gained so much weight that obesity poses as significant a health risk as smoking.

But there can be good news. Market forces will shift to meet consumer demand—manufacturers will make and sell what you will buy. Money talks, and the way you spend yours speaks loud and clear about what is important to you. Fifty years ago, African Americans pushed forward with a movement of profound social change, a stride toward freedom. By embracing a Menu for Life, we can lead America in a stride toward health and well-being. African Americans are the world's 11th largest buying power according to the 2000 edition of the annual publication, *The Buying Power of Black America.* How are you choosing to use *your* buying power?

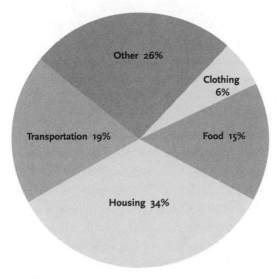

African-American Spending

THE GREAT WEIGHT MANIPULATION: SIZES LIE

Maybe you are skeptical, you think Donna and I are being dramatic about the extra pounds people are putting on and the urgency this situation creates in our African-American community as the epidemic of health problems related to obesity explodes there. A study just published in the *American Journal of Medicine* shows you have company: one-fifth of overweight patients surveyed did not know they needed to lose weight, and up to 25 percent of their doctors failed to recognize patients' weight problems. Americans have become so big, collectively, that the whole scale of our economy, our culture, our country, has shifted to accommodate how big we are.

The average African-American woman today wears a size 2X, a size that didn't exist 30 years ago. Now nearly every line of women's clothing includes some variation on plus or mature woman sizes. Large sizes—with an X or W in the label—now account for 27 percent of women's clothing sales and 15 percent of men's clothing sales. We are so big now, we need more sizes.

As weight goes up, so does clothing size. Or does it? Over the past few years, you might have noticed that even though the numbers on your bathroom scale go up, the numbers in your clothing labels stay the same, or at least increase more slowly than they used to or than you expect. When you are out shopping for clothes, this most pleasant surprise makes you feel like you are not quite so big, after all. But don't be fooled. Not only are manufacturers making bigger clothes, they are making clothes *bigger*.

The average American woman wears a size 16 dress and has a 34-inch waist. The average African-American woman's 2X dress size corresponds to a 38-inch waistline. Is it a coincidence that the average TV screen size is between 32 and 36 inches? Women's waistlines are as big as their television screens. But today's size 16 dress would have been marked a size 18 in the 1980s and a size 20 in the 1960s (the largest size on the market back then).

WOMEN'S CLOTHING SIZES THROUGH THE DECADES

1940s–1960s	1980s	2000s	WAIST SIZE
2	0	n/a	16 inches
4	2	0	18 inches
6	4	2	20 inches
8	6	4	22 inches
10	8	6	24 inches
12	10	8	26 inches
14	12	10	28 inches
16	14	12	30 inches
18	16	14	32 inches
20	18	16	34 inches
	20/1X	18	36 inches
	22/1X	20/2X	38 inches
	24/2X	22/2X	40 inches
	26/3X	24/3X	42 inches
	28/4X	26/3X	44 inches
	30/5X	28/4X	46 inches
	32/6X	30/4X	48 inches
		32/5X	50 inches
		34/5X	52 inches
		36/6X	54 inches
		38/6X	56 inches
		40/7X	58 inches
		42/7X	60 inches
		44/8X	62 inches
		46/8X	64 inches
		48/9X	68 inches
		50/10X	72 inches

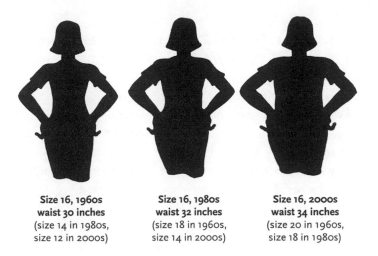

Size 16, 1960s
waist 30 inches
(size 14 in 1980s,
size 12 in 2000s)

Size 16, 1980s
waist 32 inches
(size 18 in 1960s,
size 14 in 2000s)

Size 16, 2000s
waist 34 inches
(size 20 in 1960s,
size 18 in 1980s)

Women's Clothing—What's on the Label

But, since nobody wants to watch the cashier ring up all those XXLs and 3Xs, manufacturers give us what we want to see and, more important, to buy: sizes that appear smaller than they are. The clothing industry calls this exactly what it is: *vanity sizing.* If you don't like numbers, instead of buying a 2X or a size 22, you can buy a full woman small. (Your full woman butt looks great and it is only a *small!*) An XXL, or size 48, is a big man medium. Men tend to respond favorably to big sizes, though. Go into any sports store and an XXL jersey is marketed as a symbol of athleticism and virility. The truth, most of the time, is the painful opposite.

You may think all your waist measurement tells you is what size of clothing to buy. But this simple measure actually presents a measure of your health status. When a man's waist measures more than 40 inches or a woman's more than 35 inches, there is a huge jump in the risk for heart disease and heart attack as a direct consequence of body weight. Doctors call this abdominal adiposity and now consider it a key risk factor for a number of health conditions. Though clothing sizes vary from manufacturer to manufacturer, in general a woman's size 16 to 18, or 1X, correlates to a waist measure (circumference) of 34 to 36 inches. A man's size XL correlates to a waist measure of 42 to 44 inches. If you are wearing these sizes or larger, your excess body weight gives you not only increased girth but also increased risk for type 2 diabetes, high blood pressure, and various forms of heart disease. Your weight and your health problems are directly related. Bigger bodies are not better, no matter what size is on the label. Are you a believer now?

THE PATH FROM EATING TOO MUCH TO MOVING TOO LITTLE TO WEIGHING TOO MUCH

Overeating is seldom just about food, although it might start out that way. "When I was growing up we didn't always have enough for all of us to have seconds, so often I felt deprived," says Marie Primas-Bradshaw, whose struggle with weighing too much took her from petite to plus sizes before she stabilized at a healthy weight. "When I got out on my own, I ate what I wanted and when I wanted. And when I got married, I got pregnant, I cooked, I ate, and I gained weight." Through the years Marie worked to drop extra pounds when she desired, using short-term vigorous exercise and dieting to meet specific goals like taking a trip to Europe. But the excess weight always came back. Over time, Marie realized food had become her favorite source of strength and comfort. "When I was feeling sad or lonely, when I needed nurturing, I ate," Marie says. "I was an emotional eater. I reacted to things by reaching for food rather than thinking about what kind of response I should have *for me*."

We eat for many reasons, all of us. We blame our excessive weight gain on the things that happen to us, on weight gain after pregnancy, on menopause for women or midlife for men, on an unexpected or traumatic life event such as a divorce, or caring for an aging or ill relative, or losing our job, or just because life today is too *stressful*. We eat for so many reasons other than to nourish the body, and the excess weight we accumulate as a result causes us mental and physical damage. "We have learned to eat *until* it hurts," says Stephanie Dove. "We eat until we are so full that we can't move. And then we become frustrated and unhappy, and we eat *because* we hurt, so eating becomes a source of comfort. We end up eating *all the time* so that we can feel comfort *all the time*." Food becomes emotional comfort.

"We have to learn to see food for what it is," Stephanie adds. "It is pure biological fuel. If you only eat healthy foods when you are hungry and stop when you are full, you won't overeat. It's a simple thing to do, but we make it hard for ourselves. We fail to separate food and emotion. If you want to lose weight, you have to shift your focus."

As the pounds start to pile on, people enter a cycle of obesity—a self-defeating, seemingly hopeless cycle where emotional problems and issues of daily life trigger obesity and obesity itself becomes a trigger for emotional problems. You eat because it makes you feel good when you are feeling down, makes you feel less alone. You eat more food than you need and than you should. You eat the wrong foods. You sit around the house. When you gain weight, it depresses you, disappoints you. As you get heavier, you begin to move even less because moving is more difficult because of the weight. Your activity decreases and you gain more. So you eat to feel better and lift your depression . . . and the cycle goes around and around.

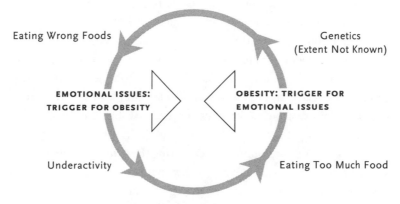

Eating Wrong Foods

Genetics
(Extent Not Known)

**EMOTIONAL ISSUES:
TRIGGER FOR OBESITY**

**OBESITY: TRIGGER FOR
EMOTIONAL ISSUES**

Underactivity

Eating Too Much Food

Cycle of Obesity

If, however, you follow the proven Menu for Life program outlined in this book, you *will* get healthy, eat well, lose weight, and live beautifully. It is working for Marie Primas-Bradshaw, for Stephanie Dove, for Cedric Williams, Alquietta Brown, Clarence White, Howard Copeland, and so many others. "When you are battling a serious weight issue and you can't seem to make any progress, you start beating up on yourself," says Marie. "You say, 'I'm fat so I might as well eat as much as I want. I'm so fat I might as well not even *try* to move around or get up off this couch.' But *you can* change yourself, *you can* control yourself. So focus there and make a start. Focus on yourself. *You can.*"

What about genetics as a way to break the cycle of obesity? Seems like every day the news is full of some new research about a hormone, chemical, or drug that either explains why we become obese or holds the promise of reducing appetite or actually dissolving fat away with a pill or prescription. Researchers do not know enough yet to apply any of these alternatives, and it may be quite some time in the future before they do. Our solution, in the meantime, takes more personal effort, and may seem in some ways old-fashioned, but it is based on the best and most current scientific knowledge we have about the process of weight gain and weight loss.

So *what is* the first step in breaking the cycle of obesity, emotional distress, and physical illness? *Stop gaining.* This is the first, and major, accomplishment. The first thing you need to do in your new Menu for Life is to learn how to stop gaining weight and bring your body's energy into a healthy balance. How do you do that? You need to take a hard, brutally honest look at how and when you eat. Bring your eating habits into the light of day where you can see and understand what it is that you are doing. When you discover how and when you eat, you can begin to see how emotion influences *your* eating. Everyone has a very personal interplay of eating habits and emotional issues. You begin to realize, as Stephanie did, that you are eating *all the time*, and for the wrong reasons. This process may not be fun or easy, but it *is* possible. Cedric could do it; so can you.

"Knowing what your habits are, separating them from emotion," Cedric says, "that's half the battle. It's not to say that you're going to kill all your habits, just avoid them until you can handle them. I don't want anyone who reads this to think they'll find a cure-all. You can't just go through life saying, no thank you. You always have to work at it. Some things, though, you just can't have anymore or do anymore. When ice cream is two for $5, I used to do that. Sit there and rationalize. I used to put the ice cream in a bowl and then said, *why?* So I just ate it from the container. Then I said, this ice cream melts, makes such a mess, *why not just eat it all?* And I did! So now, when I have to indulge I eat sorbet instead, which is healthier and has less calories. You have to figure out what you can get away with occasionally and what you need to change for good."

Let's look together at how and when you are eating.

1. When do you think about eating?
   _____ When I'm hungry.
   _____ When I see or smell food.
   _____ When it is mealtime.
   _____ All the time.
   _____ I think about food all the time when I am awake, and I dream about food when I am asleep.
2. When you last had something to eat, what was the reason that you ate?

_____ I was hungry.

_____ It was mealtime.

_____ There was too little food to save but too much to throw away after a meal.

_____ Food was there, so I ate it.

_____ I don't think about having reasons for eating.

3. Where do you keep food?

_____ In the kitchen cupboards, in the refrigerator, and in the freezer.

_____ Mostly in the kitchen, although there are bags of chips, bowls of candy, or other foods in other rooms in my house.

_____ In nearly every room of my house.

_____ In my car, in my handbag or briefcase, in my jacket pockets—just about everywhere.

4. How often do your celebrations of special occasions such as birthdays, anniversaries, graduations, weddings involve eating?

_____ Always. What's a celebration without a cake?

_____ Usually. Celebrations are times when friends and family can gather in joy and happiness, and eating is part of that.

_____ Not very often. We might have snacks.

5. When you know a special occasion is approaching (such as a wedding, graduation, or even vacation), how often do you plan to lose weight before the event?

_____ Never.

_____ When I know there will be a lot of pictures taken.

_____ When I know people will be there that I haven't seen for a long time and I want to look special.

_____ Often.

_____ Always.

6. Right now, how close are you to food?

_____ I would have to go to a store or restaurant to buy food or snacks.

_____ There is food here in my house, but I would have to prepare it.

_____ I would have to go to my kitchen to get something out of the cupboard.

_____ I would have to get something from a table in the room where I am sitting.

_____ I am eating right now, as I read.

7. When you have a meal or a snack, where do you usually eat?

    _____ I always sit at the table.

    _____ I sit at the table if there are other people eating with me, but if I'm eating alone I might stand in the kitchen or sit on the couch.

    _____ In the break room, before, during, or right after my shift at work.

    _____ I take food with me to eat while I'm doing other things, such as driving.

    _____ Wherever I happen to be when I have food, which could be at my desk, in my car, in bed, at the laundromat.

8. What was the most amount of food you ate at a single sitting, and what were the circumstances?

9. When you go out to eat, where do you go?

    _____ Fast food.

    _____ All-you-can-eat buffet.

    _____ I'd rather eat at home and fix food for myself.

    _____ I'd rather call out for food and eat at home.

    _____ A special restaurant.

10. How do you usually decide what to eat?

    _____ I think about what foods I want to eat, what I have had already to eat, and what I am planning to eat later in the day.

    _____ I look around my kitchen and choose any foods that appeal to me.

    _____ If I don't have what I want, I go to the store.

    _____ If I don't have what I want, I eat something else.

11. What kinds of foods are you likely to eat when you are in your car?

    _____ I don't usually eat when I'm in the car.

    _____ Coffee or soft drinks.

    _____ Snacks such as candy bars and chips.

    _____ Sandwiches, such as burgers, that I can eat without making too much of a mess.

    _____ Anything I might eat anywhere else.

We know that answering these questions about your eating habits honestly is a brave and difficult achievement. Yes, *achievement!* The simple act of confronting how pervasive eating is in your life and how essential eat-ing is to preserve your emotional equilibrium and sense of well-being no doubt brings up all kinds of emotional responses in you all by itself. Once you can see how the insidious cycle of obesity conspires to support your habit of overeating, you can see how obvious the need is to make some fundamental changes.

When you decide to make changes in the way that you eat, move, and live your life, you find yourself swimming against the tide of your own habits, against the tide of your loved ones and friends, against the tide of our society. No matter who you are or where you live, everyone wants you to believe that *bigger is better*. But you have eaten yourself into bigger, and you know it is not better. *"I weigh 200 pounds and I love myself*—what a crock!" Stephanie Dove asserts. "You don't love yourself when you are obese, no matter what all those people on the talk shows say."

Breaking the Cycle of Obesity

Your body is a balance of energy: Energy that you put into your body in the form of food and energy that your body expends in the form of activity. Donna and I like to look at Energy In and Energy Out as an equation:

How much you eat=Survival energy+What you do (activity)+Excess (obesity)

Every bite of food, no matter what kind of food it is, becomes energy once inside your body. Energy goes *into* your body in only one way: the food you eat. *Food Is Energy In.* When you eat too much, you give your body an *over*-supply of Energy In. Moreover, when you eat too much of the wrong foods, you give your body an oversupply of *low-quality* Energy In.

Once Energy In is inside your body it has to go somewhere. Your body takes Energy In and releases it in three ways as Energy Out.

The first energy your body uses and releases goes toward keeping you alive—what doctors call *Survival Energy*. This is the bare minimum of energy your body needs to live. Survival Energy is the energy you use to breathe and blink your eyes, to keep your heart beating, your kidneys and liver filtering, and your brain at work. When you sit around a lot watch-ing television and the only part of your body you move is your finger or thumb when you change channels with the remote, you are using little

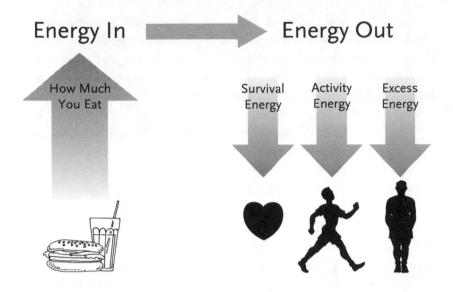

Energy In ➡ Energy Out

How Your Body Uses Energy

more than Survival Energy. That's why it is no surprise that new studies show kids who have televisions in their bedrooms or who eat in front of the television weigh more today and are more likely to become obese teenagers and adults. It takes surprisingly little food Energy In, to supply your body's Survival Energy needs.

The amount of Survival Energy your body needs is fairly constant, changing only when the amount (size) of your body changes or when other physical changes take place, such as pregnancy and aging. Pregnant women need more Survival Energy; older people need less. The more pounds you weigh, the more Survival Energy your body needs. But not that much more. Your body determines on its own how much Survival Energy it needs, without any direction or influence from you.

Energy that remains after meeting your body's Survival Energy needs becomes available for activity. Anything you do that moves a muscle, from scratching an itch to singing in the church choir to laying a new tile floor in your kitchen, uses Activity Energy. This is the energy of *what you do*. *You* control your body's Activity Energy. Whatever you do, *everything you do*, that exceeds Survival Energy uses Activity Energy. The more you do, the more active you are, the more Activity Energy you use. Activity Energy releases Energy Out. You spend the energy and it is gone as the fuel of your body in motion.

Energy that is not spent as Energy Out is stored as excess. Stored Excess Energy remains within your body in a form that is all too familiar: body fat. From the perspective of how your body functions, this energy is just as gone as if it had fueled survival or activity. Like clothes packed in boxes at the back of the closet, your body "forgets" about this Excess Energy. Even if you have days, weeks, months worth of stored Excess Energy, your body acts as though it has nothing. So you continue to take in new energy, more energy, each day, and the pounds accumulate.

To remove the Excess Energy from the Energy In/Energy Out equation, you need to *stop gaining weight*, to achieve a balance where your body's Energy In matches your body's Energy Out. When you learn to manage your Energy In by eating more healthful foods in the proper amounts and accompany this with an appropriate boost in your activity Energy Out, you achieve a balance that removes Excess Energy from the energy equation. Once Excess Energy is no longer a variable, and you succeed at reaching and holding a steady state for your weight, you can think about what you need to do to start losing pounds. But don't worry about losing weight right now. Focus on getting yourself to a steady state balance where you can comfortably and confidently keep your weight from going up. That's all you need to do to start.

Donna likes to say to people that she knows what they've been through because she's walked a mile in their shoes. And that is true. Donna has struggled with what you are struggling with. But it is more than that. Donna *knows* how to connect to what is unique and special in each person she meets. That's why her message for you now is so important, when you are at the beginning of your Menu for Life journey.

"Why do you have so little confidence in yourself?" Donna will ask you. "Because you're bombarded every day from so many sources with so many external messages telling you that you can't lose the weight. Reject negative messages. I do. Why? Because I believe in the best of myself; and I want you to believe in the best of *you*. Our people have made so much progress, our country has made so much progress, but we are being programmed to believe that *bigger is better* makes our lives easier when it does not. *Bigger is better*, when it comes to how much we weigh, is killing us. We don't need to gain any more pounds. Join us in creating a new movement—a movement toward health and well-being and living beautifully, a new Menu for Life not just for African Americans but for all of America to embrace."

3

~~~~~~~

Creating a New
Menu for Life

Sometimes, you know you need to make a change, try something new and different. Maybe you want to go back to school and get that degree you've been thinking about. Maybe you want to explore a new activity or hobby that has always interested you—painting, or learning more on the computer to earn a promotion at work, or singing jazz, or playing basketball, but you never seem to have enough time or support to fit this accomplishment into your life *right now*. Maybe you want to travel to distant places or maybe you want a few simple minutes of peace in your own backyard, but the stress of your daily schedule and the many voices shouting for your attention conspire to work against you. The man or woman in your life has one thing to say, your kids or your aging parents (or both) have their own opinions and demands, your friends push and pull you to do one thing or stay away from something else, you've got to do what you need to do at work—there's no opportunity to even *consider* yourself, though you know your own needs and desires can sit on the back burner only for so long.

Change is hard, especially when the change you need to make is a big one. And, like many things in life, one change leads to another. You realize that deciding to lose weight and to keep it off for more than a week or two involves other changes in your lifestyle and your routine that lead to still more change. How will the other people in your life respond to long-term change in you? Will they approve or disapprove of what you are doing? And, how easy will it be when you confront, head on, the conflicting, mixed messages society sends us about losing weight, about how we should look and feel about ourselves, even as we are offered the latest fad diet along with a new line of plus-sized clothing to cover it all up when the pounds come back on?

A lot of time and effort has gone into putting on those extra pounds you are carrying. It stands to reason that you'll need to put a lot of time and effort into letting them go. If someone came up to you and said they wanted to be a concert pianist and they expected to accomplish this in only a matter of months—and this person had no musical training and could barely read the notes—well, you'd probably shake your head. Donna and I know we would. If I know Donna she'd smile and tell you that line about Carnegie Hall, "the only way to get there is *practice!*" We point this out not to discourage you from your dreams, whether that dream is to be a maestro or to weigh less than you do, but to encourage you on the path of dedication and tenacity that ensures you reach your goal—no matter how long it takes, no matter what ups and downs you encounter along the way, no matter what other people (or society) have to say about your choice.

We are not talking about a quick fix, about a fad diet. We are talking about a Menu for Life, about a change for the better that becomes a lasting part of who you are and how you live. When you weigh too much— 180, 220, 270, 300, 330, or more—*there is no quick fix to lose the weight and keep it off*. At first this may seem like bad news, but it could be the best news you'll ever get for two reasons: (1) you know what you have to do, and (2) you understand that *it is possible*. And here's the best part: you will be amazed at how quickly you *do* look better and feel better, after losing only a few pounds. And ultimately you will lose as much weight *as you want to lose*, until you reach the image you want, *whatever image* looks good and feels good *to you*.

DONNA RANDALL

"I want to share with you what I am learning. What I am learning personally, *for myself*. Dealing with stress and things like that. When you look at yourself, who do *you* see? I'm only beginning to see *me*. This is what amazes me. I'm just learning who Donna is *right now*. Do *you* avoid looking in the mirror? *Why?* What is it that you are afraid of? If you force yourself to look—go ahead, *force yourself*. What do you see there? Are you looking at what other people are telling you? Are you judging before you lift your eyes to meet your own gaze? And, if so, according to *whose standards*? If looking in the mirror brings about fear, then you are not seeing *you*. You are seeing the negative of what's been heaped upon you. *And that's not you.* And that's what we have to learn.

"It is easy to fall into the trap of not knowing who and what we are when we constantly receive information about what is *ideal*. We tend to lose ourselves in our attempt to try to live up to other people's expectations of what we should be or how we should look. Too often we feel we must be or look like some *ideal*, that the person we view in the mirror has flaws, and flaws are not desirable. Let me tell you, nobody is perfect; everybody is human!

"If there is one person in the world you should want to be, you should want to love, you should want to look like, it should be *you!* I'm not selling you my ideal—for it belongs to *me alone!* No loved one, no friend, no co-worker, no talk show host, no billboard, no corporation, no person on the street can tell me what *my ideal is for myself.* And no one should pre-empt *your ideal for yourself.* If they try to do that—whether that person is your closest love or a complete stranger, politely tell them *I've got to be me!* Sometimes, the more you try to please others, the further away you get from yourself and, paradoxically, the less you seem to please anyone—most particularly *you!*

"A Menu for Life is accepting only the best for yourself, the tastes and flavors, the aroma of the world around you as you move through it and experience the joy of living and breathing and loving on this Earth. Get a good look at that person in the mirror because that person is the best friend you will ever have! Creating a Menu for Life is a decision you make from the very core of your being, and one you live every day, imperfectly sometimes maybe, but, like I said, *people are not perfect!* Everyone wants to be loved unconditionally. Give yourself this gift. Love yourself unconditionally. Create your own Menu for Life—one that is the essence of *you*, just as mine is the essence of *me*."

DR. RANDALL

"As a doctor, my focus at the hospital is on the health aspects of a Menu for Life—on helping you to make changes that will improve your health status. When you follow the Menu for Life program, you learn about the foods you are eating. You learn how to change your eating habits so you are consuming more of the right foods, while eating less food overall. You learn how important activity is to promoting the health of your body, from the inside out—your heart works better, your lungs work better, your body is healthier. As a doctor, I pay close attention to these aspects of your Menu for Life. That's my job. But the lifestyle benefits, the smaller clothes, the way you look, and the way you feel about yourself, that is health too, you know.

"There are some people who do not look in the mirror—they don't want to see who they are. They don't want to talk about it. Some people are afraid when they come into my office I will scold them about weighing some amount, I will *make* them talk about that one pound more or less. That's *not* my job. *They already know all about that one pound.* And so do you. You already know *all about* that one pound. My job is to encourage you, to safeguard your health according to my training as a cardiologist, and to educate you and give you tips and strategies to help ensure your success in getting on and staying with the Menu for Life program through all of life's ups and downs. As you read this book and explore a Menu for Life, Donna and I will give you the best of our knowledge and experience. Together we can start you moving on a path of health and well-being. Where it leads, only *you* can determine."

In medicine, we create synergy when we use different agents or actions to produce a combined effectiveness, a special benefit for the patient that is not possible or likely if we use the agents or actions in isolation. For example, if you have diabetes (type 2) you might need insulin to correct the imbalance in the way your body uses glucose, a form of sugar. You could get by just with pills or insulin injections, but if you combine insulin with adjustments in your eating and exercise habits—particularly if these adjustments result in weight loss—you can manage your diabetes more effectively. The combination of taking insulin, eating proper foods and nutrients, and losing weight can create a dynamic synergy of healthful benefit for you and perhaps reverse or eliminate your diabetes.

In life, we create synergy when we act in partnership with other people. We integrate our talents with the talents of others to produce an end result that is greater than any of us could accomplish alone. What each person contributes to the solution is unique, necessary, and beautiful—something only he or she can give. When we come out of ourselves, when we work together as a team, when we take the best of ourselves to encourage each other, we create powerful synergies for positive change in our lives, our families, and our communities. We have seen this happen again and again in our experiences in ways that continue to surprise and instruct us. We see it in the people we have met and helped through our Obesity Study—wonderful people like you. And now, we want to include you in our Menu for Life synergy of weight loss and healthy living.

OUR OBESITY STUDY: FINDING SOLUTIONS

Our Obesity Study evolved from years of observations about the apparent relationship between excess body weight and certain health problems. As a cardiologist I know firsthand, from years of treating patients who have had heart attacks, that people who have no risk factors for heart disease seldom end up looking at me from a bed in the coronary intensive care unit. I see what numerous studies confirm: that African Americans are far more likely to be in those beds than are patients of any other ethnicity. So as a physician and a researcher, I want to know how can African Americans turn these numbers around? What can you change in your life to improve your heart's health and at the same time also improve your general health status?

Other research has substantiated the increased risk African Americans face for three critical health conditions: hypertension (high blood pressure), hyperlipidemia (high blood cholesterol), and diabetes (type 2). These conditions are of deep interest to me as a cardiologist because they are the foundation for much of the heart disease that exists in the American population today. They are also conditions that we in the health care community believe we can help you prevent through lifestyle: healthful eating and regular exercise. Most people need to make lifestyle *changes.* You eat too much, and too much of the wrong foods, and you get little or no exercise. We know this because we can measure these factors, and we can measure the health consequences of these factors.

To conduct a medical study, researchers begin with a hypothesis, a statement of what you believe about what you are studying. Our Obesity Study hypothesis is simple. *Modest changes in diet and exercise can significantly improve health and reduce the risk for heart disease in people who already have one or more risk factors for heart disease.* The study is designed to collect objective data to measure the variables that surround the hypothesis. Our Obesity Study, funded by the NIH and conducted by Howard University General Clinical Research Center in Washington, D.C., had these study design elements:

- A diet of prepared meals and snacks to provide 1,800 to 2,000 calories, no more than two grams of sodium, and a distribution across food types of 60 percent carbohydrate, 25 percent fat, and 15 percent protein. This *balance* gives nearly everyone, regardless of existing health conditions, high quality Energy In.
- Moderate, sustained exercise (walking on a treadmill) for 45 to 60 minutes at least three times a week. This level of activity tones and conditions your body from the inside out, right from the cell level on up. It is intense enough to get your body to burn fat for fuel, which helps you lose stored body fat, inches, and pounds.
- Education and information about nutrition, reading food labels, choosing foods with high nutrient density, shopping, cooking, and regular physical activity and exercise. Once you know why all of these factors matter, you are better able to make decisions that benefit your health . . . without sacrificing the pleasure of eating.

Of course, in any study you need a study population—a group of people who follow the design elements so you can see what happens. For our Obesity Study our focus centered on reducing the risks of heart disease through lifestyle changes resulting in weight loss. So we selected study participants, men and women, who had:

- A strong desire to lose weight.
- A body weight at least 20 percent greater than what is healthful—a BMI of 30 or greater. This established a study population that had at least one risk factor for heart disease: *obesity.*
- Possibly one or more of these three additional risk factors for heart disease: hypertension, hyperlipidemia, or diabetes. Among the over 500 people who completed assessment for our Obesity Study, *one in two had high blood pressure, one in three had high blood cholesterol, and one in four had diabetes. One in three had two or more of these health conditions.*

We reported these findings and other study findings in the *Journal of the Academic Association of Minority Physicians.*

In a research study, it is important to control as many variables as possible. Because we knew the study's eating and exercise elements would be difficult changes for people to make, we had study participants, in small

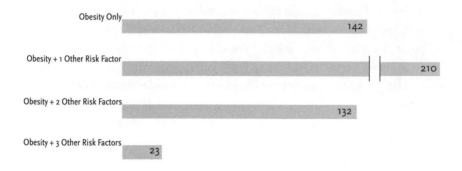

Heart Disease Risk Factors in Addition to Obesity among 507 Participants in Dr. Randall's Obesity Study

groups, spend the first week of the study in the inpatient unit of our research center. For seven days, people gave up their families, jobs, and lives. This jolted them "cold turkey" into the eating and exercise patterns we required them to follow. During this week, we measured just about everything possible that related to our hypothesis and study design, including extensive blood tests, tests for undetected factors of cardiovascular disease (such as 24-hour variability in the components of blood pressure) and kidney disease, and fat-to-muscle ratio (body composition) using the BOD-Pod pressure/volume measuring apparatus. (The BOD-Pod was interesting to study participants because it looks to many people like a body capsule from a space adventure movie!)

"I work as a nurse on the unit next to Dr. Randall's unit," says Alquietta Brown. "I heard about the Obesity Study through word of mouth and one day I dragged Dr. Randall off to the side and said, 'I *have* to get in this program! I'm 35 years old, too young to be in this shape physically, weighing over 200 pounds and needing insulin for diabetes.' Dr. Randall told me how to apply for the study and I qualified so they let me in. The *camaraderie* of the program made us all feel euphoric. Knowing you are doing things to improve your health, and exercising, which reduces stress, we all felt great."

After the first week and for the next six months, participants came to the research center at least three days a week to exercise and to pick up the meals Donna and her team prepared, meals that met the nutritional requirements we established for the study. While there, we took more measurements—weight, percentage of body fat, and waist, chest, upper arm, hip, and thigh circumferences. Here's what we found in people after only three months of their involvement:

- BMI dropped 9.7 percent.
- Weight dropped 8.5 percent (about 20 pounds for most study participants).
- The amount of body weight that came from fat dropped 17.3 percent.
- The percentage of body fat dropped 8.7 percent.

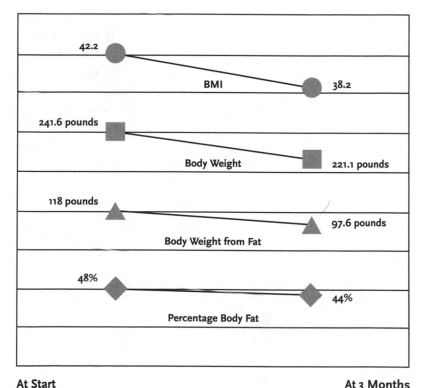

Body Composition Changes after Three Months in Dr. Randall's Obesity Study

These changes are clinically significant because they represent *major* health improvements, and are very exciting to our clinical team. Study participants found themselves excited to see the changes in their body measurements as they watched their clothing sizes drop. Most study participants went down two or three sizes in clothing. Here's how much body size decreased after only three months:

- Waist circumference decreased 7.5 percent (about three inches).
- Chest circumference decreased 5.4 percent (about three inches).
- Upper arm circumference decreased 5.2 percent (about one inch).
- Hip circumference decreased 6.3 percent (about three inches).
- Thigh circumference decreased 5.4 percent (about two inches).

From a clinical perspective, we found the decrease in waist circumference especially heartening because there is such a strong correlation between waist size and heart disease. The decrease was significant enough, in fact, that we reported it in an abstract published in the *Journal of Investigative Medicine*, Vol 50:2, p. 175A, March 2002. When exercise and diet cause a decrease in weight, BMI, and waist circumference, cardiac risk drops substantially. Study participants enjoyed the changes, too, because they felt and looked better. Best of all, as people continued to follow the study's basic guidelines for balancing Energy In and Energy Out after their participation in the study ended, *they continued to lose weight*. The study findings supported our hypothesis and our expectations, and were so

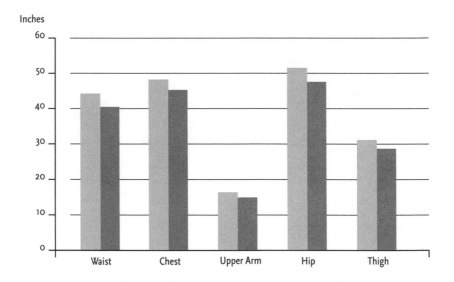

Body Measurement Changes after Three Months in
Dr. Randall's Obesity Study

compelling that they inspired Donna and me to turn our study design into a practical, easy-to-follow guide for healthy weight loss and weight management, a Menu for Life *anyone* can follow. Now through this book, we are here to partner in synergy with *you*, to help you design and develop your personal Menu for Life to meet your weight loss, weight management, and healthy living goals.

FROM STUDY TO MENU FOR LIFE

"People talk about this weight loss diet, that weight loss plan," says Stephanie Dove. "You can't live on a diet or on a plan. You have to live a lifestyle that is healthy, that is something you can enjoy. You have to live *life*." Your Menu for Life is a matter of achieving balance between your Energy In and Energy Out—what you eat and what you do—so that you can enjoy life in the ways that you want to enjoy life. How you come to this balance of Energy In and Energy Out is *your* Menu for Life. It is not mine, or Donna's, or anyone else's. It is *yours*, a Menu for Life that meets your unique needs and interests. With Menu for Life, you choose how much you want to lose, and decide where you want to maintain your weight.

When people decide to lose weight, they often have some fixed notion about what this means. Usually it means achieving a certain number of pounds lost within a specific and typically *fast* time frame. While it is good to have goals, we ask that you consider throwing away any specific goal related to your weight loss other than this one: *I want to get healthy and feel good.* While it may be highly motivating to want to get into that smaller dress or pair of pants, this should not be your primary goal. While a special event may be coming up and you want to look your best, this should not be your primary goal. While you may want to lose 100 pounds, this should not be your primary goal. While you may want to look as good as a movie star, as sleek and attractive as Halle Berry or Denzel Washington, this should not be your primary goal. We want you to give up *any preconceived ideal about your weight loss and how you accomplish it.* We want you to focus your mind and body in the here and now, in what you can do and *are doing today* to improve your health, lose weight, and feel better.

Too often, our unrealistic expectations about weight loss lead us to failure. Start small, start now, one day at a time, every day. Before you know it, you *will* see a new person in the mirror—*you!* Continue losing weight until you are happy with the image you see and then work to maintain that image—*whatever image*. Maybe you find a large butt undesirable and maybe you love a few pounds there! The important thing is being happy with the body you have and to work to make that body as fit and healthy as you can. Some things you can influence, others are out of your control. For example, if you are short and your dream is to add a foot to your height (without standing on a stepstool!), you are likely to be frustrated and disappointed in the effort to make your body do this. Similarly, your body's shape is unique to *you!* As you lose weight, enjoy seeing the *you* that emerges and forget about any cookie-cutter ideal. You are the most beautiful when you are most *yourself!*

"I'm 200 pounds now," says Cedric Williams. "I was down to 190 for a while, but I decided I looked too thin there. I'm satisfied at 200, comfortable at 200, even though the model says I should weigh 170. Now I work to maintain that. Maintenance, in some ways, is more important than losing! Losing, you dedicate yourself and watch the results. Maintenance can be more elusive, but from day to day there is real pleasure in knowing your efforts are supporting your health. So maintenance is not really hard. I thought it would be much harder than it is."

The framework for Menu for Life is simple and follows the same guidelines we established for our Obesity Study to balance Energy In and Energy Out while providing your body with the nutrition and exercise that it needs to function at its best. These are the basic components of Menu for Life:

GIVE YOUR BODY HIGH-QUALITY ENERGY IN

- Eat 1,800 to 2,400 calories a day of nutrient-dense foods that you enjoy.
- Get 60 percent of your daily calories from carbohydrate, 15 percent from protein, and 25 percent from fat.
- Limit your daily intake of sodium to 2,000 milligrams.

You must eat enough. You need to eat an adequate amount of food to meet your body's energy and health needs. When you fail to do so (as in fad diets that severely restrict your calories as Energy In), your body compensates in ways that compromise your vitality. You feel weak and tired because your body is not receiving adequate nutrition. We know, after years of extensive research, that the human body needs a minimum of about 1,800 calories worth of Energy In, in the appropriate ratio of energy sources, to supply it with the energy and the nutrients it needs. We also know that only professional athletes, dancers, and others who push their bodies to their physical limitations on a regular basis need to eat more than 2,400 calories a day. Our Menu for Life meal planner shows you how to plan meals, a week at a time, around nutrient-dense foods that keep you feeling full and satisfied—giving options for daily calorie targets of 1,800, 2,100, and 2,400 so you can choose the level that best meets your needs.

You must eat the right kinds of foods. In your Menu for Life, you should get 60 percent of your Energy In from carbohydrate, 15 percent from protein, and 25 percent from fat. Here's why we believe this is the right balance for nearly everyone:

- We know that just over half of the functions of living that take place within your cells every day require glucose for fuel—this is the *only* fuel your brain, nerve, and red blood cells can use, and is the fuel muscle cells use when they first move into action. Based on this knowledge we tell you, *get 60 percent of your Energy In from dietary carbohydrates.*
- We know your body dedicates about 10 to 12 percent of its functions to repairing and building cells and tissues. Amino acids are the core building materials it needs to do this, and we know that dietary protein provides your body with the energy source it needs to generate amino acids. Your body must receive certain amino acids directly from the foods you eat and it can manufacture other amino acids it needs from these amino acids and from other substances. Based on this knowledge, and to make sure you cover your body's needs for essential amino acids, we tell you, *get 15 percent of your Energy In from dietary proteins.*
- We know your body uses lipids, the forms fat takes within your body, for a number of important functions including transporting certain vitamins and as fuel for muscle and other cells during sustained activity. From our knowledge about how your body uses fatty acids, we can tell you *get about 25 percent of your Energy In from dietary fat.*

You must consume less sodium. Nearly all Americans get too much sodium; sodium appears in nearly all fast foods, prepared foods, canned goods, and processed foods. Plus we use salt (which is 40 percent sodium) as a seasoning. A diet high in sodium contributes to high blood pressure. Your Menu for Life gives you 2,000 milligrams of sodium a day, more than enough to meet your body's needs and your taste desires for salt. We tell you how to use other seasonings to develop a taste for more various and interesting flavors.

GIVE YOUR BODY HIGH-QUALITY ENERGY OUT

- Get your body moving!
- Look for opportunities to increase your physical activity through regular functions of everyday living.
- Get 30 for 5—at least 30 to 45 minutes of sustained exercise 5 days a week.

Your body needs to move. We all spend far too much time sitting still, letting our bodies do hardly even the bare minimum. Get moving! No matter what you are doing, there are ways to make it more active, more physical—to increase your Energy Out. "Put on the clothes you find comfortable and just get moving," says Marie Primas-Bradshaw. "You want the weight off! Then you can put on the spandex or whatever cute things you want to wear."

Make every day active. What kinds of things do you *do* each day? There are countless ways to increase your activity level. We will show you how to explore your day to find these opportunities, to look at the time you spend doing nothing or being inactive, and find ways to use this time for your benefit and enjoyment.

A little regular exercise delivers significant health benefits. Your body needs regular, sustained (continuous) physical activity—moderate exercise—to keep it functioning at its best, and to keep your heart, and your body, healthy and strong. We know from numerous studies (including our own Obesity Study) that it takes only a little effort to get a lot of benefit: just 30 to 45 minutes of moderate exercise 5 days a week, physical activity that gets your heart pumping and your lungs expanding. Walking is the easiest way for most people to meet this level of activity. But you can walk, run, swim, bike, dance, do yoga or t'ai chi, play sports—whatever you *like* to do.

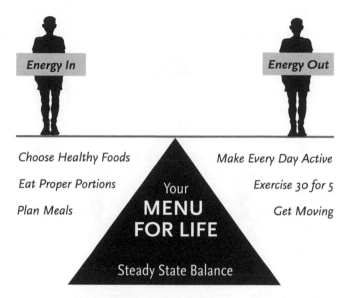

We had our Obesity Study participants make a clean break from their old habits. This approach might work for you. Or you may want to make more gradual changes. Start anywhere you can. Start where you are, because wherever you are is just fine. If you eat 5,000 calories a day right now, drop 500 calories or 1,000 calories a day until you are comfortable with the 2,400 calorie target we suggest. You will still lose weight, especially if you are also increasing your activity and getting exercise. It is more important to do this slow deduction in daily calories than to start out with the unrealistic expectation of going directly from a higher amount of calories to 1,800 or 2,100 calories a day and then not being able to do it, or to stick with it. What is important is to have a lifestyle that is acceptable, that you *will follow*, over a long period of time. Start walking whenever you have the opportunity, even if that means marching in place in front of your television set at first. You will feel better. *You will lose weight.*

When your Energy In and your Energy Out are in balance, your health is in balance. Your life is in balance. So, first: *stop gaining.* When you stop gaining, you work to achieve a steady state balance. Then: *start losing weight.* When you reach the weight you want, work to maintain that weight by continuing to eat correctly and by staying with your exercise.

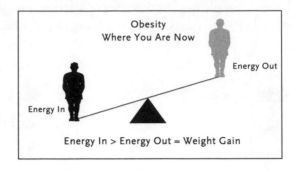

Obesity
Where You Are Now

Energy Out

Energy In

Energy In > Energy Out = Weight Gain

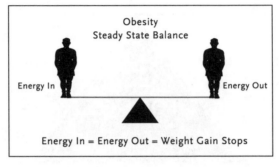

Obesity
Steady State Balance

Energy In

Energy Out

Energy In = Energy Out = Weight Gain Stops

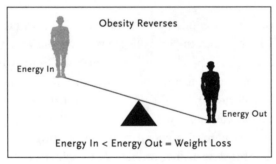

Obesity Reverses

Energy In

Energy Out

Energy In < Energy Out = Weight Loss

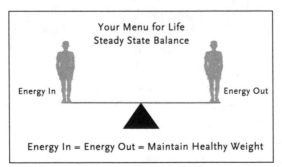

Your Menu for Life
Steady State Balance

Energy In

Energy Out

Energy In = Energy Out = Maintain Healthy Weight

From Obesity to Maintaining Healthy Weight

Have you seen your doctor in the last year? When you weigh too much you might feel reluctant to see a doctor unless you absolutely have to. Or if a health condition related to your weight is a reason you are reading this book, you might be seeing too much of your doctor. In either case, schedule an appointment with your doctor specifically to talk about your interest in losing weight. Let your doctor identify any health issues you need to accommodate as you develop your Menu for Life. The Menu for Life meal planner is designed so that you can easily address whatever special nutritional requirements your doctor may give you to enhance your health. Do you have health problems that make exercise difficult or challenging? Your doctor can help you figure out what you can do that you enjoy. No matter what your physical constraints or present fitness level, you can become more active. Take this book with you for your appointment, so your doctor can see what you are doing and can become an active partner in your efforts and your progress.

"I recently had some ankle surgery," says Howard Copeland, "so I needed to find something else to do besides the treadmill. At first I couldn't get around much at all and I put back some weight. I got bored too, you see everything that's on the television and then you get impatient to be back moving again. I'm starting on the stationary bike now with my physical therapy. I prefer the treadmill, but since I can't do that right now, I'll try this for a while. The first time I rode it 20 minutes, but I hurt my leg so now I'm only doing 10 minutes and working my way back up. I'm doing wonderfully and I'm determined to stay with it."

CREATING YOUR MENU FOR LIFE

We are creatures of habit. We do the things we do, eat the foods we eat, because we do. We always have, at least for as long as we can remember. This is what we *know*, so it is what we *do*. With Menu for Life, we are going to give you new knowledge, new ways of looking at what and how you eat and exercise, to help you establish new habits, habits that support your good health. You are used to preparing foods in certain ways, and to the ways those foods taste and make you feel when you eat them. What is your favorite food? Why is it your favorite? How long has it been your favorite? The foods we like best are often ones we have been eating for longer than we can remember. Do you love fried fish because you love fried fish, or because this is how you have always eaten fish? You might say because you love it fried. But when was the last time you ate fish prepared any other way?

Take a few minutes right now to write down the foods you must have:

FAVORITE FOOD	HOW MUCH OF IT I EAT	HOW OFTEN I EAT IT	HOW I FEEL WHEN I EAT THIS FOOD

Donna and I will never ask you to give up *any* of these favorites. You may have to eat less of them, and eat them less often. You may have to find different ways to prepare and enjoy some of them (and Donna will show you how) so that these favorites are healthier for you, but they will remain part of your life.

Most Americans eat too much fat and sugar—not through conscious choices or because they are following diets that instruct them to, but because it is just the way they eat. How often do you eat fast food? If you eat fast food three times a week or more, you eat too much fat and sugar! Most Americans eat at least twice as much food as their bodies need, and many eat three to four times as much.

Knowing *when* to eat is as important as knowing *what* to eat and *how much* to eat. The problem today is: *we eat all the time.* Many of us even eat in our cars! No matter where you go, there is food—at work, at school, at celebrations. When you eat all the time, it's hard to know how much you eat. When you start eating the right foods, you feel full for longer. It takes less to satisfy you, because what you are eating is meeting your body's nutritional energy needs.

Take a look at how African Americans are spending their food dollars. We spend more on fats and sweets than on fruits and vegetables combined! In Chapter 8, you will learn how to rebalance your plate so that you are getting the correct percentages of energy sources from the foods you eat. Guaranteed, once you do that, you will begin to spend your food dollars more wisely. How wonderful it would be to see the Menu for Life movement take hold, and watch those spending patterns move toward more healthful food choices.

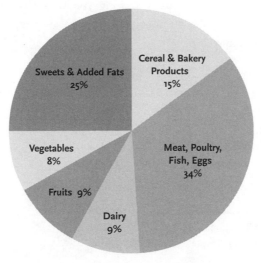

How African Americans Spend Their Food Dollars

One in three African-American men and one in two African-American women—half!—*get no physical activity at all*. What activities do you like to do? Do you like to walk? Walking is a great activity, and it can be terrific exercise. Look for ways during your day to become a little more active, ways to give your body a little more to do. This can be as simple as using a manual can opener instead of an electric one! Opportunities are all around you. Take a few minutes now to write down activities and exercise you enjoy, or that you used to enjoy:

Activity or Exercise That I Enjoy	How Often I Do It	How Often I Could Do It If I Planned It	Any Reasons That I Can't Do This Activity or Exercise

Regular physical activity *must* be combined with healthful changes in eating habits—eating the right foods in the correct portion sizes—to achieve balance in the Energy In/Energy Out equation. If you continue eating as you eat now, look at how long you would have to walk at a moderate pace (three miles an hour) to balance the Energy In provided by the foods listed below:

FOOD (ENERGY IN)	TIME WALKING TO BALANCE (ENERGY OUT)
KFC chicken breast, original recipe	1 hour, 40 minutes
KFC chicken breast, extra crispy	2 hours
Skinless chicken breast, broiled at home	35 minutes
Long John Silver battered and fried fish, 1 piece	1 hour
Long John Silver flatbread fish sandwich	3 hours, 5 minutes
McDonald's Big Mac	2 hours, 30 minutes
McDonald's Quarter Pounder with Cheese	2 hours, 15 minutes
Burger King Double Bacon Cheeseburger	2 hours, 25 minutes
Burger King Whopper with Cheese	3 hours, 40 minutes
Pizza Hut Stuffed Crust Meat Lover's, 1 slice of large pizza	2 hours
Denny's Original Grand Slam Breakfast	4 hours, 15 minutes
Taco Bell Taco Supreme	1 hour, 5 minutes
Taco Bell Mucho Grande Nachos	5 hours, 30 minutes
Small fries	55 minutes
Supersize fries	1 hour, 50 minutes
Soft drink, 20-ounce (not diet)	1 hour
7-Eleven Double Gulp	3 hours, 20 minutes
Pecan pie (1/6 of 8" pie)	1 hour, 40 minutes
Krispy Kreme doughnut, glazed ring	50 minutes
Large apple	15 minutes

"I don't ever plan to get over 200 pounds again," says Clarence White, "and with Menu for Life I have the right plan to do that by eating right and exercising. My ideal weight would be 190, but I go up, I go down. I weigh myself every now and then, and I take my own blood pressure with a machine in the morning and the evening. Menu for Life is not a complicated process when you think about it. Get rid of the sodium, get rid of the sugar, get rid of the grease, and exercise. Watch the portions that you eat. Cooking for yourself is best. I don't think it can be any simpler than that. It's a way of life for me now."

WHAT *DOESN'T* WORK IN A MENU FOR LIFE

What you may *really* like to do is take a pill and not get fat, or take a pill and lose weight. Someday researchers might make this fantasy reality, but even if it works, that pill is unlikely to address the needs your body has to eat nutritiously and to move. *Your body needs to eat and move!* The next best thing to a pill, then (so goes the logic), would be a fad diet. While some of these fad diets may be put together in ways that are more or less healthful, most are skewed in an unhealthy way for short-term weight loss. You need a Menu for Life that is something you can do—and something *you will want to do*—that is healthful for you *every day for the rest of your life.*

Americans spend $5 billion a year on weight-loss products and services that are outright frauds. Powdered drinks or supplements that "dissolve" fat while you sleep. Devices that stimulate muscle contractions to "burn" fat while you watch television. *These products do not work*, plain and simple. But we buy them, because we are willing to try *anything* to lose weight. Don't let promises of a "miraculous new discovery" or a "magical ancient secret" lure you into spending your money—and wasting your precious health. If these products really worked, how many people do you think would still weigh too much?

Even legitimate weight-loss medications, ones your doctor might prescribe for you, have no direct effect on your weight or your body fat. Instead, they influence your desire to eat. When your urge to eat is suppressed, it is easier to resist eating and to comply with a regulated food intake. As long as you take the drug you feel full and satisfied to eat smaller amounts of food, and to eat less frequently. But you can't take these drugs forever. Many of the drugs are new and researchers are still exploring their side effects, both short- and long-term. Once you stop taking the drug, once the chemical "gatekeeper" is gone, your appetite is no longer artificially suppressed and most people return to their previous eating habits and resume gaining weight.

When your body gets to weigh *a lot* too much, you feel desperate to make changes. In recent years, new surgical procedures make it possible for people to lose vast amounts of weight in relatively short periods of time. These are solutions of last resort. The potential side effects post-surgery are serious and long-term. Gastric reduction surgery shrinks the stomach's standard holding capacity of 50 to 70 ounces to a mere 4 to 6 ounces, barely 10 percent of its natural design. This surgery forces weight loss because it reduces the amount needed to fill your stomach! At first, this may seem great to you, but think about it. You love to eat, and you *should*. Eating healthfully is a primary goal in a Menu for Life. If you have gastric surgery, you will never again be able to eat and enjoy food as a normal, healthy person does. You will struggle to get enough nutrients to nourish your body appropriately. And, though your stomach will no longer hold the food, that does not mean you will lose your desire to eat. If you follow our Menu for Life, you can enjoy your food *and* lose the weight without putting your body through an extreme surgical procedure. For most people, gastric reduction surgery is a dangerous desperate solution with far more down sides for the long term than up sides for the short term.

What *Does* Work in a Menu for Life

A true Menu for Life is one that, as it takes form, endures and grows. As the days and weeks pass, when you look in the mirror you will see that your determination is paying off in ways you may not have anticipated when you started, but that you delight in now. As you lose inches and pounds, your confidence grows. You know you are doing the right things when you focus on eating healthfully and getting your sustained exercise. You look better. You feel better. You are acting from a centered sense of being that grows stronger and stronger within you. Sure, you will have setbacks. Let them make you stronger too by surviving them. Be motivated by these words from WNBA All-Star Teresa Weatherspoon, "I believe in doing whatever it takes to move an obstacle. I don't believe there is anything in front of me that can stop me from getting to where I want to be. I've always been that way."

A Menu for Life is something you share. When the people around you see what you are doing and understand that you are doing your Menu for Life for the long haul, for the *rest* of your life, your example will inspire and instruct *them*. More than your accomplishments or failures, others will see and champion your stamina, devotion, and dedication to sticking with your Menu for Life. We think it's safe to say that on your Menu for Life journey you will find a buddy who will want to join you. And that's great. Look for this person and nurture and support each other every day.

We need to do this, be this kind of model, especially, for our families and our children. If we fail to act now, today's generation of overweight children will become tomorrow's generation of obese adults. Already we see children with health problems children should not have. Heart disease is unnatural to a child. Diabetes (type 2) is unnatural to a child. *Obesity* is unnatural to a child. You need to lead the way, for your *own* health, and for your family's health.

"What you are really doing when you do your Menu for Life is this: *you are loving yourself*," Donna says. When you read this book and work to educate yourself about your health, about how to lose weight and keep it off, you unlock the door to understanding. Once you unlock one door others open before you—compassion, hope, peace, community, health.

"Because we are unique in ourselves, we each have something special to give to each other, to teach each other. We are creating a beautiful synergy. I can grow from that. You can grow from that. Together, we pass our knowledge on to others, and in turn, we open ourselves to learn from them. Dr. Randall and I want you to know that is what all of this is about—a rich, full Menu for Life that celebrates healthful eating and engages you in life's activities shared with the people you love."

Part Two

~~~~

How Less Is More!

4

～～～～

Energy In: How a Body
Gets to Weigh Too Much

Your body weighs too much. You see it when you glance in the mirror or when you catch your reflection in a window. You see it in the expressions of other people who, whether they stare at your body or look away quickly, rarely make eye contact with you or hold your gaze. No matter how much care you take to dress in a way that hides how big your body looks, it is still big. Your weight is causing you noticeable problems. Problems finding clothes that fit. Problems fitting into the seats in restaurants and movie theaters. Problems wearing seat belts. Problems, too, with your health: health problems that become increasingly severe, increasingly difficult to ignore, increasingly distressing. But still, you gain *more* weight. You might even joke that all you have to do is *look* at food and you gain five pounds.

What gives? Surely, this fat man or fat woman couldn't possibly be you. *I'm not that fat person; I don't look like that. That can't be me.* Your reflection surprises you all too often. The weight of the truth takes your breath away, and you know you are foolish to ignore the heaviness anymore. Maybe you have had enough (we hope so!); you are ready to stop gaining and achieve a steady state for your weight, a major accomplishment. You are eager to take a deep breath in and begin work on your new Menu for Life.

In this chapter, we're going to take a look at the left half of the Energy In/Energy Out equation: Energy In, or, HOW MUCH YOU EAT. The reason you weigh so much is deceptively simple in most cases: you feed your body too much. You don't mean to do it, and you might not even realize how much food is too much food. But the fact is: *You give your body more food than it needs.* In the Energy In/Energy Out equation, your Energy In far exceeds your Energy Out. With nowhere to send all that extra energy (extra food), it becomes body fat on the other side of the equation.

We're going to talk to you about what happens in your body when you eat too much, the physiology of weight gain. Knowing how and why your body gains weight helps you understand how to bring your body's energy back into balance. We will explain what led you to where you are now . . . as well as help you to see where you want to be, and how to get there from here.

DONNA RANDALL

"There is only one way to put energy into your body: you eat it. A lot of overeating comes from stress, depression, things like that, and you have got to learn how to keep the out-of-control eating from sending *you* out of control. If you recognize what you are doing, then, when someone asks you, 'why are you overeating?' if you say you don't know why, you're in denial. We want you to tune in and start addressing your situation in a positive way. We want to help you put your eating, your Energy In, into healthy balance with your Energy Out."

DR. RANDALL

"You need to start first by thinking about how much food you eat. If you eat a smaller amount of whatever it is that you are eating, you will lose weight. But here is the *real* challenge and joy: to eat less food, while getting to think more creatively about eating, about variety, nutrient density, and all the things Donna will tell you about. That is why portion control, smart food choices, and following the Menu for Life program are so important. I believe it is *more enjoyable*, because eating is such a favorite activity, to *think* about it, to be more creative about what you eat, and to have fun with healthier choices. You will still feel full, but it will be a healthier full. Why do you weigh too much? Because you eat too much. Because you have too much energy going in to balance the amount of energy you have going out. And you eat the things that are least healthy for you, in quantities that are far too large. It doesn't have to be that way. You can change."

The Energy In/Energy Out equation describes metabolism: the process through which energy becomes available to your body. We know from Chapter 2 that energy goes in (the food you eat) and that energy—in countless forms of activity from basic breathing to strenuous exercise—

comes out. But there is much that we *don't* know about what happens in between, and this unknown is the key for researchers in the future to understand how to manage weight. Until we learn more about what goes on inside this "black box" of metabolism, all that we can do is manage what we already understand: Energy In and Energy Out.

Although the scientific discussion of metabolism is complex and detailed, metabolism is simply the actions that take place starting with Energy In (eating) and concluding with Energy Out (activity). When Energy In dominates, you are in a state of *anabolism*. When Energy Out dominates, then you are in a state of *catabolism*.

Anabolism + Catabolism = Metabolism

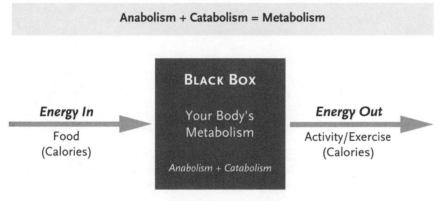

The "Black Box" of Metabolism

Everyone's metabolism is different; your metabolism is unique to you. Metabolism knows no race or ethnicity. No one really knows why metabolic efficiency varies among individuals, and it is this variability that makes weight gain and weight loss so different from person to person. Menu for Life is about maximizing your personal metabolic efficiency to find the right balance. When you reach a steady state, in which there is harmony between Energy In and Energy Out, your weight remains stable. To get to a point of weight loss, catabolism must exceed anabolism until you obtain your desired image. Then, lock in at the new steady state where Energy In equals Energy Out.

In metabolic terms, quick weight-loss diets often attempt to force weight loss by severely restricting your Energy In, while making no changes to your Energy Out. But this leads to metabolic *unbalance* and provides an unhealthy, unsustainable solution to the energy equation. If the solution were that easy, quick weight-loss diets would work for everyone. And we know, through experience, that they don't! True weight loss comes from decreasing Energy In appropriately while increasing Energy Out appropriately for maximum health benefits. And when you find the weight that is right for you, you maintain your steady state balance.

Often we talk about metabolism in terms of "fast" or "slow." We all know people who can eat anything without gaining an ounce and other people who gain weight rapidly without eating very much. We blame a "slow" metabolism for weight gain or inability to lose weight and credit a "fast" metabolism with weight loss or preventing weight gain. Certainly there are many scientific variables in the ways your cells use energy. Whether your metabolism is "fast" or "slow," by adjusting the equation to take less Energy In, your cells redirect their efforts from storage—making fat—to supplying the energy output your body needs to fuel its activities as you increase movement, breathe, and live.

How Food Becomes Energy

Calories aren't news to you. Every diet you have ever tried made you count them. But do you *really* know what a calorie is or why calories matter? There is a technical, scientific definition, of course, that leaves even doctors scratching their heads! But in the end, a calorie is just a measure of energy. Not of food, but of energy. A calorie is a value, not an amount. Even though we look at foods in terms of the caloric values

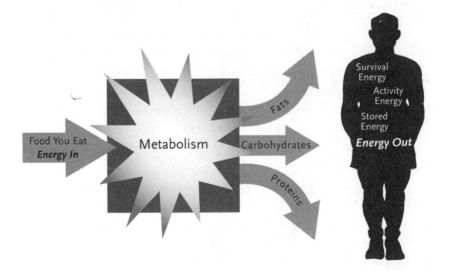

From Food to Energy Sources

they contain, you can't see, touch, taste, or smell a calorie. Foods have different caloric values:

Type	Calories per Gram	Calories per Ounce	Sources	Examples
Carbohydrate	4	120	sugars, starches, soluble fiber	table sugar, fruits, potatoes
Protein	4	120	animal-based foods, certain legumes	meats (steak, ham, poultry, etc.), fish, eggs, cheese, butter, soybeans
Fat	9	270	animal-based foods, dairy products, nuts, avocados, processed foods, vegetable oils	red meats and poultry with skin, olive oil, milk, eggs, cashews, cheese, baked goods, desserts
Alcohol	7	7	alcoholic beverages	wine, cocktails, beer

Carbohydrate, protein, and fat are the main energy sources your body's black box of metabolism uses from the foods you eat, your Energy In, to fuel your Energy Out.

To your body, a calorie is a calorie is a calorie. Inside the black box of metabolism, it no longer matters where the calorie comes from. One calorie from a chocolate chip cookie has the same *energy value* as one calorie from an apple. But bite for bite, the chocolate chip cookie delivers more calories because the source for some of its calories is fat. Look at this comparison:

	Apple 3 1/4 inch diameter	Chocolate Chip Cookie 3 1/2 inch diameter
Protein Calories (4 calories per gram)	0	2 grams = 8 calories
Carbohydrate Calories (4 calories per gram)	32 grams = 128 calories	27 grams = 108 calories
Fat Calories (9 calories per gram)	0	9 grams = 81 calories
Total Calories	128	197

For all its energy value, fat is much lighter both as a substance and nutritionally. Foods that are low in dietary fat such as fruits, vegetables, and grains (including rice, breads, and cereals) have higher nutritional density than high-fat foods like cake, cookies, and chips. There is actually a one-two benefit in eating such low-fat nutrient-dense foods. One: you feel fuller for longer after eating these foods, *because* they are nutritionally dense. Two: not only do they deliver fewer calories (less energy), but also you *feel full faster* when you are eating, so you tend not to eat as much.

"Main meal" foods that are high in fat that you might be eating now, such as fried fish or fried chicken, do stick with you longer than "snack" kinds of foods that are high in fat, primarily because the fish or chicken is also high in protein (which takes longer for your body to digest). But even when the balance between protein and fat is even in terms of weight, it is greatly unbalanced in terms of calories—every gram of fat contains more than twice as many calories as every gram of protein. Fat in the foods that you eat "supersizes" Energy In. And with nowhere to go if you are inactive, this energy "sits down" and becomes body fat. It is much easier for your body to convert dietary fat into body fat than to convert dietary protein or carbohydrate into body fat.

The flip side: by volume, body fat weighs less than any other substance in your body. If you could take a gallon of fat from our body, it would weigh about a third to half as much as a gallon of muscle. So when you are losing inches, you are losing body fat—*even if it doesn't appear that you are losing much weight.* This paradox of fat—double the energy, half the weight—explains why you can lose inches quickly but it might be slower to lose pounds. You are losing weight when you lose inches, even if it doesn't seem so.

Just as importantly, when you lose body fat, you take pressure off your body in ways the scale just can't measure. Excess body fat puts pressure on all of your body's organ systems, interfering with their abilities to function at their maximum and best potential: respiratory, cardiovascular (circulatory), digestive, and others. Being obese puts an incredible strain on *every* function of your body. And when this "too much excess" body fat accumulates around your belly—what we call abdominal adiposity—your risk for heart disease shoots skyward.

How a Body Gains Weight

You gained weight bite by bite, pound by pound, day by day, year by year. You can probably look back to a time (or at pictures of yourself) when your weight was healthy. When was that time? What do you remember about it? More likely than not, you were more active then. You played sports, went dancing, even just went out walking. "I never weighed more than 140 pounds in all my life," says Alquietta Brown. "Then in 1993 I got out of the military and stopped being active. But I kept eating like I was still active. My weight shot up and all of a sudden I weighed 210."

While she was in the military, Alquietta exercised regularly. Staying fit was a job requirement, and exercise formed as much a part of her daily routine as putting on the uniform. When Alquietta got out of the service, her lifestyle changed. She could wear what she wanted, and no one cared whether she stayed fit or not. She stopped exercising. But she didn't stop eating. Alquietta continued to eat as she'd grown accustomed to during her military career, but with no outlet for all of the energy this eating increased her body mass. So her weight crept up, a pound or two a month, until after five years she found that her body had grown perilously close to being twice the size it had been when she left military service. And with the weight gain came a sudden and serious consequence: diabetes.

A registered nurse, Alquietta knew her diabetes diagnosis meant that her life had taken a dramatic new direction. But she also recognized she could still make decisions to put her life back on a healthy path. "It took getting sick for it to bother me to be fat," Alquietta recalls. "I could buy all kinds of fancy clothes to look like I wasn't as fat as I was. I knew I was fat, but I just dressed it up! But then I got sick, and I knew I *had* to do something about my weight, and I *wanted* to do it."

This is how most people get the message that they weigh too much—something goes wrong with their bodies. Just 35 years old when her doctor gave her the bad news that she had diabetes and needed to start taking daily insulin shots, Alquietta made changes to get her body to a healthy weight and improve her health. Following the Menu for Life approach, Alquietta lost 60 pounds and has kept the weight off, with a few little ups and downs. She looks and feels great, has plenty of energy for her busy family and career, and no longer shops for clothes that hide her body. Best of all, Alquietta says, "My blood sugar now is normal!"

When people talk to Donna and me about how they got to weigh so much, they almost always point to specific life events and circumstances: pregnancy, getting married, menopause, getting divorced, getting a new job, losing a job, having a child move away from home, having an adult child move back home, stopping smoking, getting out of college, getting out of the military, not playing sports anymore, middle age, caring for aging relatives. The reasons for gaining weight are as diverse as individual people are! We've heard them all and lived through more than one of them as a couple over the years ourselves. In the most primal sense, when you feed your body, that physical nourishment *feels* emotionally satisfying too. When you have a lot of stress in your life, you need *extra* nourishing, body and soul. And when you need extra nourishing, you may turn to emotional eating in a desperate attempt to find it—quickly, and in the largest quantity you can.

"Understand the connections between stress, emotion, and eating," Donna says, "and once you can see these connections you can target your stress and release it in other ways—yoga, exercise, music, reading, gardening. Anything that helps you redirect the energy of your emotions out to constructive and positive alternatives is good. Because, you see, we're back again to energy. Stress *feels* like Energy Out, which leads you to want to increase your Energy In. But you don't have to cope with it that way! You can learn healthier ways to deal with and reduce stress. Learning to eat the right foods in the right quantities is one of them! You don't have to swallow your stress—which creates more stress on top of the stress you *already* have because you are eating too much of the wrong foods. Instead of reducing your stress and making you feel emotionally and physically better, you gain *more* stress and *more* pounds and *more* pounds and *more* stress, as your emotional eating leads your Energy In farther and farther out of balance."

"If you are putting more Energy In because of emotions, you can't reach balance," says Marie Primas-Bradshaw, who lost 40 pounds during her participation in the Obesity Study. "I was good at blaming other people and other things for making me so upset that I ate. But then I had to tell myself, 'You bent your elbow and put that food in your mouth!' Once I accepted that, I could make changes."

We want you to learn to look at food for what it is—the energy that fuels your body's functions and activities. In a true Menu for Life, you nourish your body with healthy, wholesome foods and you nourish your soul by moving and living to the fullest! You are the embodiment of Energy In and Energy Out. The balance of metabolism is *your* balance.

COULD IT BE GENETIC?

In 1994, researchers reported the exciting news that they had isolated an "obesity gene." The timing of their discovery coincided with our awareness that more people than ever were overweight or obese. It wasn't just that individuals weighed more; the *entire* average had crept up toward the point where the average itself began to fall into the zone of unhealthy. The hypothesis that genetic influences could be at work in obesity suggested to researchers that there might be other ways to approach weight management.

Further studies have shown that the obesity gene appears to play a role in the release of chemicals in the body that signal the brain's appetite center. When this gene is defective (or mutated, as doctors say), it allows the brain's appetite center to send signals that the body interprets as "Eat!" even when the stomach is full and the body's nutritional needs are met. Further research also showed that despite appearances that obesity runs in families, a defect involving this gene is *extraordinarily rare*. It is highly unlikely that you weigh too much because of genetics.

Genetics actually play a very, very small role in body weight. Body style and shape, yes—your genetic makeup influences, and even regulates, your physical appearance. But body style and shape are *not* the same as body weight. It might run in your family that when you do put on weight, it gathers in your thighs, on your hips, in your arms, or around your belly. These are familiar patterns linked to the genes that determine your body structure—in the same way that your genes determine how much hair you have on your arms and legs. They are *not* patterns of genetic fatness. With extremely rare exceptions, you accumulate excess body fat and weight because your Energy In exceeds your Energy Out.

The obesity increase that we have witnessed over the last 30 years is clearly a consequence of behavior changes. We eat more and exercise less. A change in gene structure takes many generations, not just a few decades, to manifest. If there is an obesity gene, it has been there all along . . . we just haven't been feeding it! Even when we look at the higher rates of obesity in certain ethnic groups—for example, nearly seven in ten

African-American women are overweight—the reasons relate to lifestyle, not to genetics or to ethnicity.

You don't weigh more because of an obesity gene. You weigh what you do because of the ways you eat and exercise. Although it would be much easier to find the answer to the question, "Why do I weigh too much?" in science because then the situation truly is out of your control, the truth lies much closer to home—it is within you. And this is good news! In fact, it's the best news possible, because it means that *you can change.*

MEASURING OBESITY

When you get right down to it, you don't need a scale, a tape measure, or even a mirror. You know that when your clothes have an "X" or a "W" on the label, your body is too big. A bigger body tells your doctor, before knowing anything else about you, what health conditions to check you for. So why bother to measure your weight?

Not so long ago, doctors used height/weight charts to determine whether a person's body weight was "average" or "normal." These charts listed all kinds of variables—height, age, small bone structure, medium bone structure, large bone structure, male, female. You could pretty much pick and choose to find the category most favorable for you. You could say, "Well, I've got big bones," and gain yourself an extra 20 pounds or so of "acceptable" weight.

These charts didn't really show doctors the correlations between body weight and health. Instead, they were actuarial charts—one of the many tools that life insurance companies used to determine a person's risk of dying. People whose weight was within the appropriate category had a "no greater than average" chance of dying prematurely—that is, of dying earlier than the typical life expectancy based on birth date. When your weight fell outside the appropriate category, so did your risk for dying young. You became more of a liability for the life insurance company, which charged you more for insurance because of it. Doctors borrowed these charts to provide a structure for looking at body weight as a health factor because at the time they had no other tools to use.

What we know now is that most of the variables these height/weight charts incorporated don't really matter when it comes to assessing the risk that body weight contributes to health—not even gender and age. We now know that if your weight is in the correct range for your height your risk for health problems is no greater than average. When your weight is beyond the healthy range, your risks for health problems go up. The further from the healthy range that your weight is, the higher your risks are until you reach a point where you are certain to have health problems *because* of your weight, not any other factor. The tool that represents the degree of risk is the BMI. The easiest way to find your BMI is to use the BMI chart on page 76, which gives you a whole number figure as your BMI.

BMI is so much more valuable than the old height/weight tables because it makes the connections between body weight and health problems very clear. BMI represents your body mass in kilograms per meter squared, which you often see written as kg/m² (kilograms per meter squared). BMI is derived from a mathematical formula that converts height and weight figures into a scale of values rated according to potential health risk. The correlations come from years of medical research and analysis. To find your precise BMI, which is more useful in assessing your personal health risks related to weight, you need to do a little math. For all numbers, round to the nearest tenth. Here's how you do it:

- Weigh yourself (without clothes). For our two examples here, we will use 150 pounds and 280 pounds.
- Measure your height (without shoes) in inches. For example, 5 feet 4 inches equals 64 inches; 6 feet equals 72 inches.
- Multiply your height in inches by itself: 64 x 64 = 4096; 72 x 72 = 5184. This is your height in inches squared.
- Divide your weight in pounds by your height in inches squared: 150 pounds ÷ 4096 = 0.037; 280 pounds ÷ 5180 = 0.054.
- Multiply the result by 704.5 (the conversion factor to give you kilograms per meter squared): 0.037 x 704.5 = 26.1kg≠m²; 0.054 x 704.5 = 38.026.1kg≠m².

A BMI over 25 is overweight. For most people, this represents a body weight that is about 10 percent greater than it should be. When your BMI passes 30, your body fat is about 20 percent more than it should be—the point of obesity. (Over 90 percent of adults with type 2 diabetes are obese.) And when BMI goes over 40, it is unusual *not* to have health problems

BODY MASS INDEX (BMI) CHART

BMI	19	20	21	22	23	24	25	26	27	28	29	30	31	32	33	34
HEIGHT (INCHES)							WEIGHT IN POUNDS									
58	91	96	100	105	110	115	119	124	129	134	138	143	148	153	158	162
59	94	99	104	109	114	119	124	128	133	138	143	148	153	158	163	168
60	97	102	107	112	118	123	128	133	138	143	148	153	158	163	168	174
61	100	106	111	116	122	127	132	137	143	148	153	158	164	169	174	180
62	104	109	115	120	126	131	136	142	147	153	158	164	169	175	180	186
63	107	113	118	124	130	135	141	146	152	158	163	169	175	180	186	191
64	110	116	122	128	134	140	145	151	157	163	169	174	180	186	192	197
65	114	120	126	132	138	144	150	156	162	168	174	180	186	192	198	204
66	118	124	130	136	142	148	155	161	167	173	179	186	192	198	204	210
67	121	127	134	140	146	153	159	166	172	178	185	191	198	204	211	217
68	125	131	138	144	151	158	164	171	177	184	190	197	203	210	216	223
69	128	135	142	149	155	162	169	176	182	189	196	203	209	216	223	230
70	132	139	146	153	160	167	174	181	188	195	202	209	216	222	229	236
71	136	143	150	157	165	172	179	186	193	200	208	215	222	229	238	243
72	140	147	154	162	169	177	184	191	199	206	213	221	228	235	242	250
73	144	151	159	166	174	182	189	197	204	212	219	227	235	242	250	257
74	148	155	163	171	179	186	194	202	210	218	225	233	241	249	256	264
75	152	160	168	176	184	192	200	208	216	224	232	240	248	256	264	272
76	156	164	172	180	189	197	205	213	221	230	238	248	254	263	271	279

BMI	35	36	37	38	39	40	41	42	43	44	45	46	47	48	49	50
HEIGHT (INCHES)							WEIGHT IN POUNDS									
58	167	172	177	181	186	191	196	201	205	210	215	220	224	229	234	239
59	173	178	183	188	193	198	203	208	212	217	222	227	232	237	242	247
60	179	184	189	194	199	204	209	215	220	225	230	235	240	245	250	255
61	185	190	195	201	206	211	217	222	227	232	238	243	248	254	259	264
62	191	196	202	207	213	218	224	229	235	240	246	251	255	262	267	273
63	197	203	208	214	220	225	231	237	242	248	254	259	265	270	278	282
64	204	209	215	221	227	232	238	244	250	256	262	267	273	279	285	291
65	210	216	222	228	234	240	246	252	258	264	270	276	282	288	294	300
66	216	223	229	235	241	247	253	260	266	272	278	284	291	297	303	309
67	223	230	236	242	249	255	261	268	274	280	287	293	299	306	312	319
68	230	236	243	249	256	262	269	278	282	289	295	302	308	315	322	328
69	236	243	250	257	263	270	277	284	291	297	304	311	318	324	331	338
70	243	250	257	264	271	278	285	292	299	306	313	320	327	334	341	348
71	250	257	265	272	279	286	293	301	308	315	322	329	338	343	351	358
72	258	265	272	279	287	294	302	309	316	324	331	338	346	353	361	368
73	265	272	280	288	295	302	310	318	325	333	340	348	355	363	371	378
74	272	280	287	295	303	311	319	326	334	342	350	358	365	373	381	389
75	279	287	295	303	311	319	327	335	343	351	359	367	375	383	391	399
76	287	295	304	312	320	328	336	344	353	361	369	377	385	394	402	410

Adapted from National Institutes of Health, National Heart, Lung, and Blood Institute (NIH/NHLBI)

THE BODY MASS INDEX (BMI Scale in kg/m²)

IF YOUR BMI IS . . .	THEN YOUR WEIGHT IS . . .	AND YOUR HEALTH RISK IS . . .
18.5 to 24.9	Healthy	Not affected by your weight.
25.0 to 29.9	Overweight	Increased for heart disease, high blood pressure, insulin resistance syndrome, diabetes (type 2), and some forms of cancer.
30.0 to 34.9	Obese—Class I (Moderate)	Increased for coronary heart disease (CHD), congestive heart failure (CHF), diabetes (type 2), certain cancers, osteoarthritis, sleep apnea, and gallstones.
35.0 to 39.9	Obese—Class II (Serious)	Significantly increased for CHD, CHF, high blood pressure, heart attack, stroke, certain cancers, diabetes, osteoarthritis, sleep apnea, gallstones, kidney disease as a complication of diabetes and high blood pressure, and premature death. Women also are at increased risk for infertility, menstrual cycle irregularity, polycystic ovary syndrome, and complications during pregnancy.
40.0 or higher	Obese—Class III (Extreme)	Likely to have significant, multiple health problems including CHD, CHF, high blood pressure, certain cancers, insulin-dependent diabetes (type 2), osteoarthritis, sleep apnea, and gallstones, with significantly increased risk for heart attack, stroke, kidney disease, and kidney failure, and premature death.

directly related to body weight. The chart shows how BMI values correlate to weight and health risk.

A BMI over 30 is associated with a big increase, three to four times that with a BMI under 30, for high blood pressure, high blood cholesterol, and diabetes—the building blocks of heart disease, kidney disease, and stroke. These health conditions are the leading causes of death in the United States. Your health risks continue to increase as your BMI rises. From the "big three" health risks (diabetes, high blood pressure, and high blood cholesterol) extend the paths to the diseases that kill us: heart disease, kidney disease, stroke, and even some kinds of cancer. If you are African American, your risks are exponentially higher—we know this to be true, although we don't know entirely why.

When your weight gets to a BMI over 40, no amount of medical treatment can make you better again until, and unless, you lose weight. This is the point at which your weight becomes a critical factor in health problems of all kinds, from those we just mentioned to other conditions such as arthritis (excess weight increases the strain on your joints). This is not a judgment of you or your lifestyle or your willpower or any of the other mental traps or mind games that go with weighing too much. It is not about how you look or the clothes you wear or how much room you take up when you sit on the couch. It is, pure and simple, a medical reality.

How Much Do *You* Eat?
Your Portion Size Profile

So, how much *do* you eat? How do you *know* how much you eat? For many people, the answer to both questions is, "I don't know." That's okay, because within the next few pages you will learn, or at least you will begin to have a pretty good idea. And you *need* to know. You need to know how much you eat so you can see how much energy you are putting into your body. You need to know how much you eat so you can begin to make choices that better support your health and happiness.

So let's take a look at what you are putting on your plate and into your mouth. Here are some questions to help you measure *how much* you eat (not what, but simply how much). Be honest with (and kind to) yourself. There are no right or wrong answers. All you are doing is identifying how much you eat right now, so you can plan your path to where you want to be. Before you can start losing, you have to stop gaining.

1. How often do you eat?
   _____ Three times a day—breakfast, lunch, supper
   _____ Two times a day—I skip breakfast or lunch
   _____ One time a day—I skip breakfast and lunch and eat a big supper
   _____ Every two hours or so, snacks and meals combined
   _____ I always have food of some kind in my hand
2. What size (diameter) is the plate you use for your main meal of the day?

_____ 12 inches

_____ 10 inches

_____ 8 inches

3. How much do the glasses that you usually use for serving beverages hold?

_____ 6 ounces

_____ 8 ounces

_____ 12 ounces

_____ 16 ounces

_____ 20 ounces

4. How often do you have more than one helping?

_____ Just about every meal

_____ When it's my favorite food

_____ When it's a special meal, like Thanksgiving

_____ If what's left over isn't enough to save but would be wasteful to throw away

_____ To make the cook feel good

_____ Seldom or never

5. When you pour yourself a glass of milk, juice, soda, or other beverage, do you:

_____ Look at the label to see what a serving size is and measure that amount

_____ Splash enough in the glass to quench your thirst

_____ Fill the glass

_____ Fill the glass to the brim, take a drink, and top it off

_____ Drink from the container

6. When you have cereal for breakfast, do you:

_____ Look at the cereal's label to see what a serving size is and measure that amount and then look at the label on the milk carton and measure that amount

_____ Fill the bowl to the top, then pour on the milk

_____ Eat from the bag or box

7. When you want a snack, do you:

_____ Look at the label to see what a serving size is and measure that amount

_____ Grab a handful

_____ Pour some into a bowl

_____ Eat right from the package

8a. When you go out for pizza with your significant other, what do you order?

_____ Individual-size pizzas . . . just cheese

_____ Individual-size pizzas . . . everything

_____ One medium-size pizza . . . just cheese

_____ One medium-size pizza . . . everything

_____ One medium-size pizza . . . double everything

_____ One large-size pizza . . . just cheese

_____ One large-size pizza . . . everything

_____ One large-size pizza . . . double everything

_____ One super-large pizza . . . just cheese

_____ One super-large pizza . . . everything

_____ One super-large pizza . . . double everything

8b. How much pizza do you usually take home with you?

_____ Half

_____ A fourth

_____ A slice or two

_____ None

9. When you stop for fast food, what do you order?

_____ A regular sandwich and a small drink

_____ A small combination meal (regular sandwich, fries, drink)

_____ A "supersize" combination meal (large sandwich, large fries, large drink)

_____ A combination meal that includes two small meals (2 sandwiches, 2 fries, 2 drinks)

_____ Two or more meals of any kind

10. At mealtimes at home, do you:

_____ Put each food item in a serving dish and place the serving dishes on the table

_____ Fill your plate from the cooking dishes, and sit at the table to eat

_____ Fill your plate from the cooking dishes, sampling as you go, and stand in the kitchen to eat

_____ Sometimes put food on a plate, sometimes eat from the pan or cooking dish

11. When you go out for dinner with friends, how long before you leave do you have something to eat?

_____ The previous meal

_____ An hour or two

_____ Less than 30 minutes

_____ Right before leaving

12. How many servings are in a 20-ounce bag of chips?

_____ 20

_____ 10

_____ 5

_____ 1

When you are eating too much, the serving sizes listed on food labels seem ridiculously small. And for you they are, because you are used to eating much more. If you look at the nutritional information on any food item, from a bag of peanuts to a carton of milk, you will see an * (asterisk) at the top of the chart. This links you to the fine print that says, "Percent Daily Values (DV) are based on a 2,000-calorie diet." This is how many calories a "standard" person requires in a day to support a moderate level of activity (some labels list values for 2,000- and 2,500-calorie diets).

When the amount of food that you typically eat is equal to two or three times the serving size on the label, you are probably eating two to three times as many calories in a day overall. So instead of that 2,000-calorie or 2,500-calorie intake that is the "standard," your Energy In is 4,000 to 5,000 calories or more a day. It doesn't seem like that much to you because you are used to eating that way. But when you start to list it out, you become uncomfortably aware of just how much you eat. Denial will slow down or stop your progress: *To thine own self be true!* A Menu for Life is for the *rest* of your life, and your family's too. Face what you eat daily and how much. You cannot conquer the unseen enemy. You owe it to yourself to come out of this battle as a conquering hero! Go over the list again, and be sure your answers are accurate. You may find that just coming clean to yourself about how much you really eat is enough to help make a change.

PORTION SIZE OR SERVING SIZE?

Portion and serving sizes are the key to understanding how much is enough. A portion size is the amount of food that you actually *do* eat. A serving size is the amount of food that is nutritionally appropriate. Are you surprised at how much you eat during a typical day? Most people are.

When you eat too much, the portions you have become accustomed to as normal are often two to four times as big as a suggested serving size. How long does a 20-ounce bag of chips last at your house? The label says there are 20 servings in that bag—and that each serving contains approximately six chips. If you are used to pouring half the bag into a bowl or eating straight from the bag, you really have no idea how much you eat although you can be certain it is much more than one serving.

With beverages, too, you often don't realize that you pour yourself the equivalent of three or four servings. You just want a glass of milk or a bottle of soda! The label on a 20-ounce bottle of soda typically says "2.5

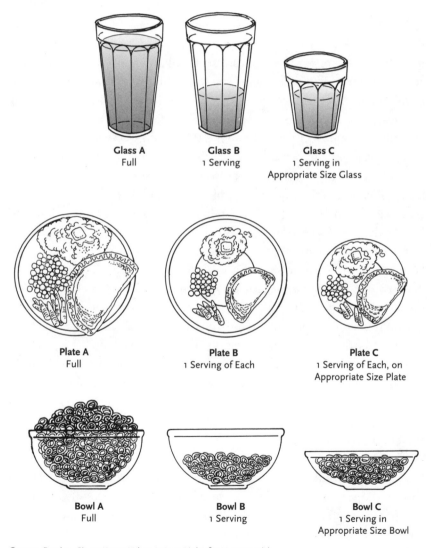

Glass A Full	**Glass B** 1 Serving	**Glass C** 1 Serving in Appropriate Size Glass
Plate A Full	**Plate B** 1 Serving of Each	**Plate C** 1 Serving of Each, on Appropriate Size Plate
Bowl A Full	**Bowl B** 1 Serving	**Bowl C** 1 Serving in Appropriate Size Bowl

Correct Portion Sizes: Know What Is Just Right for Your Health servings." (Twenty or thirty years ago, the standard-sized bottle contained only 6 or 8 fluid ounces.) One serving from the 20-ounce soda bottle is listed as 8 fluid ounces. If the calorie value per soda serving is 100 calories, when you drink the whole 20-ounce bottle (as most of us are tempted to do), you are getting 250 calories—not 100! The 20-ounce bottle may seem like more value for your money, but if you drink it all at once, you get less value *for your health!*

You may want to counter this with: *Why can't I drink a whole 20-ounce bottle of diet soda, which contains 0 calories?* There's sodium in that diet soda (not good if you have hypertension), a lot of chemicals, and, like regular soda, not much nutritional value. If you want to quench your thirst, the healthiest beverage you can drink is water. And water contains 0 calories. Drink as much water as you want, as often as you can. Be careful, though, about bottled waters fortified with flavors and other substances that may add as many as 100 calories or more. Leave diet soda on the grocery store shelf.

Here are some suggestions to help you make better choices when it comes to bringing your portion sizes closer to appropriate serving sizes:

- Read labels. What is the serving size? Measure it out so you can see what it looks like on your plate, in your bowl, in your glass or cup. How does it compare to what you usually eat? Serving sizes are often one-third to one-half of what you think . . . and what you usually take.
- Use dishes that are the appropriate sizes for the foods you are eating and their serving sizes. This is partly a matter of psychology; if the food on your plate looks like it fills your plate, you feel more satisfied about the amounts you are eating. But it is more a matter of practicality because it helps you to see what appropriate, healthy servings look like—and to choose them. And it is not just your plate. A typical drinking glass holds 12 to 16 ounces, yet a typical serving size is 6 to 8 ounces. Fill your too-big glass and you give yourself the equivalent of two to three servings.
- Take only what you need to meet your body's nutritional requirements. If you are an emotional eater, this gives you confidence because you are in control. And when you are confident, and managing your eating, you are not at the mercy of what is on your plate!
- Make a photocopy of the diagram on page 82 and post it on your refrigerator as a visual reminder of correct (healthy!) portion sizes.

Your Menu for Life: Balancing Energy In

When you first recognize that you eat too much, it can shock you. Facing reality is sometimes like that, just like when you go to the doctor and the doctor tells you that your blood pressure is up and you need to start taking medication to bring it under control. You need to make different choices so you can start managing the energy that you put into your body to bring Energy In into healthy balance. Right now, we want you to look at what, and how much, you eat. Focus on the portion sizes of the foods you eat, and begin to examine how many calories come from dietary fat. Eating less, but healthier foods is something different from starving yourself, or giving up all of your favorite foods. Remember, if you are eating 5,000 calories a day and you eat only 500 calories less, you will lose weight. The change in the amount and type of food you eat does not have to be dramatic to yield dramatic health benefits.

Listen to Donna: "You need to make lifestyle changes, yes. But these are not changes of sacrifice. These are changes of control, choice, and health. And once you start making these changes, you will be *amazed* at how good you feel. Dr. Randall and I don't want you to stop eating food; we want you to stop *gaining pounds*. We want you to *change* the way you eat and the way you *think* about eating. We want you to sit down to a low-calorie, low-sodium meal that is so nutritionally dense that you can't finish it—and yet that is so flavorful and satisfying that you feel fulfilled. *This* is your Menu for Life."

5

~~~~~~

Weighed Down
by Health Problems

*T*hrough the years, as your body gets bigger, your mind gets used to it. This convinces you that your body gets used to it too. Your mind lets you believe that even though your body is big, it is still healthy. You tell yourself you can be fit and be fat. You can carry the weight and be healthy. You look good. Why make such a fuss about extra pounds? Extra pounds may slow you down but not so much that you feel they deserve so much attention. Besides you made your peace with those extra pounds long ago, and you suspect, whether you are happy about it or not (and we guess you are not), those extra pounds are here to stay. You may have an aunt or uncle who has diabetes or a friend with high blood pressure, but that's not you. Or, if it is you, well, then, what does that diabetes or high blood pressure have to do with gaining weight?

Over the years, your body has been sending you messages and signals—little things nagging for your attention, but your mind is a great and creative force that interprets these warnings in ways that reassure you. That your knees hurt before you step from your bed onto the floor in the morning, that's just morning creakiness. That bending over to reach your feet to tie your shoes is difficult if not impossible to do, well you gave up training for the Olympics years ago! That you get short of breath walking down the steps—those steps are *steep*. But deep down you sense these messages are telling you something more, something you want to ignore as long as you can because you fear there may not be anything you can do. These signals and messages—doctors would call them symptoms—are common when you weigh too much; they tell you your body is struggling to support your weight. Can you carry the weight, be fit and fat, be fat and healthy? No, we believe the answer is no.

Let's start with a closer look at the symptoms we just talked about: your bones ache and creak in the morning, you are unable to bend down and touch your toes, you get short of breath quickly in situations where you probably should be able to breathe without difficulty. Under the burden of the extra weight your feet have to carry, the tendons and ligaments that support your bones begin to stretch and lose flexibility. When your BMI passes 30, the point of obesity, the structure of your feet flattens under the pressure of your body weight. When you look at the footprint you leave on the bathmat when you step out of the shower or tub, it is full. There is no distinct, curved line to the outside, with a firm heel print and clear toe prints on either end. There is just one big, elongated oval.

This tells you the tendons and ligaments of your foot, of your arch, are worn and stretched, and they no longer hold you up as they should. Your ankles, your knees, your hips, your back, even your neck—all change to compensate. Your body pulls itself into an unnatural alignment as it works to accommodate the strain. These are the changes your body makes to carry and balance your excess weight, and they are the changes that eventually cause damage because they force your body away from its intended design. Your once-in-a-while aches and pains become deep, chronic joint pain. Meanwhile, your mind lets you believe the changes have no significance. This is simply the way it is.

DONNA RANDALL

"Every now and then the brothers come out and walk with me. *Osteo* and *rheumatoid*. You know: *arthritis*. Oh, and their cousin, *bursitis* too! This trio does a lot of traveling, so probably you have met them too. They certainly came to visit me the day the publisher shot the photograph for the cover of this book. Through two wardrobe changes and several hours I stood with Dr. Randall while the photographer snapped away taking picture after picture. In the down time when the photographer changed a lens and checked the lighting, I decided not to focus on my aches and pains but to entertain everyone with my rendition of a Pearl Bailey standard. Dr. Randall and I love jazz and we were having so much fun, and that's the moment you see captured on the cover. I wish I could come right over to your house and sing your aches and pains away. Moving, eating right—the right foods in the correct portion sizes—enjoying life with the people closest to you, that's all part of a Menu for Life. When you take care of yourself, when you do the things that promote your health and well-being, you look and feel beautiful. That's right, honey. We're smiling *at you!* Tell the trio to head for the hills and start doing your Menu for Life. Your aches and pains will ease up for you, and chances are good you'll feel more like singing too."

DR. RANDALL

"You can look at a Menu for Life in a lot of different ways. One way is to look at it as secondary prevention. This means you are doing your Menu for Life because you have already had a health problem, such as a heart attack, so now you want to lower your weight, lower your cholesterol to help your heart. That's *secondary* prevention. *Secondary* prevention, you've had a major health problem, and you want to decrease the chances of it happening again or continuing. But, if you haven't had a heart attack, and you weigh too much, have high cholesterol, and, let's say you smoke too, doing your Menu for Life is primary prevention. *Primary* prevention is when you have only the *risk factors* that *may* lead to a disease. You want to stop the risk factors in order to avoid the disease. Obesity itself is an independent risk factor. Whether your purpose is primary or secondary prevention, avoid obesity and you reduce your risk of hypertension, diabetes (type 2), and hyperlipidemia.

"Did you know the number one cause for the alarming increase in diabetes (type 2) in this country is obesity? Among African Americans the diagnosis of diabetes (type 2) has increased almost four times since 1968, and we have to believe that today, when two in five African-American women and two in ten African-American men are obese, that weighing too much is a strong contributing factor in this increase of diabetes. Did you know that a five to seven pound weight loss yields a 58 percent decrease in cardiac complications from diabetes—things like coronary artery disease and atherosclerosis? We don't know whether this trend continues as you lose more weight, but the main point is that this small weight loss produces greater health benefit than we in the medical community hoped to find. So subtract five or seven pounds from whatever it is that you weigh now, and you accomplish something *very important* for your health.

"But there is another kind of prevention we never talk about—you don't even have the risk factors, and you want to prevent them from coming. So, avoid making that transition from overweight to obesity! *Stop gaining weight.* Watch your BMI (go back and take another look at the chart in Chapter 1) and make sure it stays under 30. *Avoid obesity altogether.*

"All of the research we are doing on obesity and its impact on health problems is important knowledge for the medical community in waking doctors and other health care professionals up to the current epidemic of obesity, and how to deal with the rising epidemic of the consequences of obesity. But, well, we've known a lot of things for years about the health problems associated with weighing too much and still people are eating and not moving and gaining pounds! So we want to talk to you, one on one, about what decisions you are making about your health, about your *life*, when you chose to keep eating too much, when you chose to stop moving, when you keep putting on the pounds.

"Donna and I believe that once you fully understand the risks associated with weighing too much, then weighing too much will not be something you resign yourself to, that you accept, any longer. You will not want to do it anymore. You reach a steady state balance where you avoid adding any more weight, and then you begin to lose weight at a safe and healthy pace using your Menu for Life, and you keep the weight off. We've helped hundreds of people accomplish this. As Donna says, doing your Menu for Life becomes something you do for the joy of life. *Your life.* We want you to have a long and happy one!"

What size shoe did you wear when you were at your prime, in your best physical condition, at your lowest weight? What size and *width* do you wear today? "I always had cute little feet, so I could wear nice shoes," says Marie Primas-Bradshaw. "Even when I had to wear bigger clothes, I still could wear nice shoes. Then my feet started getting bigger. I had to go to wide widths, and I had to say, 'okay, *now* I have to change.' It was part pride, but also part realizing that this weight affected all of me. I was gaining weight everywhere and feeling it right down to my feet."

As long as you weigh too much, health problems get worse, and they cause other health problems. It becomes a spiral of sorts, one thing that leads to another to another to another. Every cell feels the effects. Your breathing ability diminishes, your arteries become less resilient, your muscles lose tone and mass. Your circulation is not as good as it could be, especially if you also have diabetes. Your weight even affects your body's ability to resist illness and to heal, so you seem to catch every little virus that comes along and to be down with it longer than other people. Other health problems have the opportunity to develop . . . and they do. "I had some problems with sleep apnea with my weight gain," says Howard Copeland. "One night my daughter heard me struggling to breathe and woke me up. We thought I was having a bad dream, but the doctor said it was sleep apnea, that I stop breathing when I'm asleep." Being too heavy causes or contributes to many health problems, minor and major. Some of these problems—such as sleep apnea and gastroesophageal reflux disorder (GERD), that acid feeling that repeats on you and that you can feel when you lie down in bed or on the couch—usually go away entirely when you lose weight. Other health problems are more significant, and once they gain critical mass, once they establish a firm presence in your body, their consequences are more significant and may become permanent.

The changes that you do see and feel tell you that changes you may be unable to see or to feel are taking place within your body as well. Nearly 13 percent of all African Americans have diabetes. According to the National Diabetes Information Clearinghouse, "about one-third of total diabetes cases are undiagnosed among African Americans." *Undiagnosed.* Fifty million Americans have hypertension, or high blood pressure, a condition often called "the silent killer" because while it does damage inside your body there are no overt external signs and symptoms you can see or feel. To know you have high blood pressure, your doctor has to take blood pressure readings. Only half the people who have high blood pressure are aware that they have it! Of those who are aware, only half of them are receiving treatment. And of those, only half of them have their blood pressure under control (blood pressure less than 140/90). So, of those 50 million Americans, 37.5 million are still at significant risk for complications from hypertension.

Hypertension occurs in men, women, old, young, black and white, rich or poor, but it occurs most often in African Americans. It starts at a younger age and reaches a higher level in a shorter period of time, is more difficult to control, and African Americans have more complications from it. The reasons for all of these differences are unknown. But we do know that obesity increases your risk for both diabetes (type 2) and hypertension. Seeing your doctor regularly and taking medications as prescribed are only part of the answer. You also need to take care of your life through diet and exercise—your Menu for Life.

The signs are there for your doctor to read. Sometimes, though, your doctor tells you that you are heading for a health crisis unless you get your weight under control. But your mind still convinces you that you are really fine, that maybe the doctor is trying to scare you. "I was always the big one in my family," says Cedric Williams. "And I wasn't just big, I was *very* big! My doctor told me all the problems my weight was causing me but I didn't listen. I've had hypertension since I was 38, then I got diabetes and congestive heart failure. I was on medication for all of them, and that made me feel safe. I ate like I wanted to, never got off the couch, and I kept getting bigger. I weighed over 350 pounds, and one Saturday morning the right side of my body quit working. I was 42 years old, and I had a stroke."

Weighing too much, eating too much of the wrong foods, moving too little—these circumstances set the stage for three major health conditions. We'll discuss all of these in greater depth later in this chapter, but for now here is a quick snapshot of each: high blood pressure, high blood cholesterol, and diabetes (type 2).

- HIGH BLOOD PRESSURE (HYPERTENSION). When the pressure in your blood vessels increases, as happens when you gain weight, it takes more effort for your heart to move it through your arteries. High blood pressure is the leading cause of stroke and kidney disease, including kidney failure. These conditions affect African Americans more frequently and more severely.
- HIGH BLOOD CHOLESTEROL (HYPERLIPIDEMIA). Multiple factors contribute to high levels of lipids and fatty acids in the bloodstream that then build up along the walls of the arteries. High blood cholesterol contributes to high blood pressure by narrowing and stiffening your arteries, making your heart pump harder to move blood through them. The deposits of lipids that collect along your artery walls can break loose under the increased pressure, causing heart attack and stroke.
- DIABETES (TYPE 2). High blood sugar identifies diabetes, but diabetes is a disease of insulin dysfunction. When you have diabetes (type 2), your body is not properly responding to insulin or is not making enough insulin. In the intricate balance of your body's chemistry, this affects many body functions including how your body metabolizes lipids. Heart disease is a major and common complication from diabetes.

There is a *direct and measurable connection* between your weight, obesity, and these health conditions. In Chapter 4 you identified your BMI. This number is important for what it tells you about your weight and also for what it tells you about your health. Your risk for health problems rises with your BMI. When your BMI reaches 28, approaching the upper limits of overweight, your risk for diabetes (type 2) is already three to four times that of someone of healthy weight whose BMI is 25 or under, and you are twice as likely to have high blood pressure. When your BMI reaches 30, the official point of obesity, you are certain to have at least one mild to moderate health problem that is related to your weight, most likely high blood pressure—at a BMI of 30 or higher, one in three women and two in five men have high blood pressure, a reading of 140/90 or higher. When your BMI goes over 35, serious obesity, you are fairly certain to have more than one health problem. You are more likely than not to have high blood pressure. You might have high blood cholesterol. You likely have high blood sugar (glucose), indicating early stage or full-blown diabetes (type 2).

When your BMI goes over 40, the clinical term for your condition is *extremely obese. Your health problems directly threaten your life.* Doctors used to call this condition "morbid obesity"—the point at which your weight is such a strain on your body that it can no longer function properly, the point at which your risk of dying *doubles* as a direct and sole consequence of your weight. When your weight becomes such a significant factor in your health, doctors are often powerless to fix the many problems that result. Under these circumstances, all doctors may be able to do is to treat conditions in a way that delays their consequences. Only *you* can lead yourself back to better health. And you *can* lead yourself to better health. As soon as you *stop gaining* weight, you take a giant leap forward. When you start *losing* weight, every pound that you lose improves your health. *Every* pound lost counts for better health.

YOUR BMI AND HEALTH RISK

BMI	HEALTH RISK BECAUSE OF YOUR WEIGHT	HEALTH PROBLEMS RELATED TO YOUR WEIGHT THAT YOU LIKELY ALREADY HAVE	HEALTH PROBLEMS FOR WHICH YOUR RISK INCREASES
18.5 to 24.9 **Healthy weight**	**None**	none related to weight	none related to weight
25 to 29.9 **Overweight**	**Elevated** two to three times more likely to have health problems than with a BMI under 25	mild high blood pressure, insulin resistance	high blood pressure, insulin resistance, diabetes (type 2)
30 to 34.9 **Obesity** 15 to 25 percent above healthy weight	**High** one or two mild to moderate health problems related to your weight	mild high blood pressure, insulin resistance, mild arthritis, mildly elevated blood cholesterol	high blood pressure, diabetes (type 2), arthritis, high blood cholesterol, heart disease, gallstones, sleep apnea, some cancers
35 to 39.9 **Serious Obesity** 35 to 45 percent above healthy weight	**Probable** two or more health problems related to your weight that require medication	high blood pressure, high blood cholesterol, diabetes (type 2) requiring medication; sleep apnea; arthritis that restricts your physical activity	high blood pressure, coronary artery disease, stroke, diabetes (type 2) requiring medication, arthritis, sleep apnea, gallstones, kidney disease, some cancers, premature death
40 and above **Extreme Obesity** body weight is half again or more above healthy weight	**Certain** multiple health problems related to your weight that require treatment and that interfere with activities you enjoy	high blood pressure, high blood cholesterol that require one or more medications each; diabetes (type 2) that requires insulin shots; sleep apnea; arthritis that restricts your physical activity; congestive heart failure and other heart conditions that require medication	high blood pressure, congestive heart failure, coronary artery disease, heart attack, stroke, diabetes (type 2), arthritis, sleep apnea, gallstones, kidney failure, some cancers, premature death

When Cedric entered our Obesity Study he had a BMI of 48. He lost 50 pounds during his six months in the study—a rate of about 2 pounds a week that brought his BMI down to a much-improved but still at-risk 41.

Over the following three years, Cedric lost another 100 pounds, dropping his BMI to a much healthier 27. Today, he follows the Menu for Life Energy In/Energy Out guidelines to maintain a steady state for his weight and his health. "I hate to think that somebody would have to go through what I did," says Cedric. "But I did it to myself. *You* don't have to do it to *yourself*. I hope someone can read this and say, 'I can do this. I can change before I have a stroke or this or that happens.' I want you to know, you don't have to go down the same route that I did. You can break the cycle of obesity and health problems, before it breaks you."

YOUR PERSONAL HEALTH RISKS

The best place to start is with an understanding of what health problems you may already have and which health problems are a particular risk for you because of your personal or family health history. The answers to these 20 questions can give you a clearer picture of how your weight is affecting your health and how changes that you make in your lifestyle can improve your health status. Come back to these questions as you implement your Menu for Life, to see how the numbers may change. Write your responses here in your book or photocopy these pages to keep the information separate.

1. What is your height?
2. What is your weight?
3. What is a healthy weight and BMI for your height (The range of healthy weights for your height, can be found in the BMI table in Chapter 4.)?
4. What is your BMI (Calculate from the table on page 75 in Chapter 4.)?
5. What is your health risk based on your BMI (Find this on the table on page 77 in Chapter 4.)?
6. For what health conditions are you at increased risk?
7. What is your blood pressure?
8. When did you last have your blood pressure checked?
9. Do you currently take medication for your blood pressure?
10. Does anyone in your family (parents, brothers, sisters) have high blood pressure?

11. What are your blood cholesterol levels?

_____ Total cholesterol

_____ HDL

_____ LDL

_____ Total-to-HDL ratio

12. When did you last have your blood cholesterol levels checked?

13. Do you currently take medication to lower your blood cholesterol?

14. Have you had a heart attack or stroke?

15. Have any members of your immediate family (parents, brothers, sisters) died of heart disease before age 55?

16. Have any members of your immediate family (parents, brothers, sisters) had a heart attack or stroke before age 55?

17. Do you have high blood sugar, prediabetes, glucose intolerance, or diabetes?

18. Are you taking medication for diabetes?

19. Does anyone in your family (parents, brothers, sisters) have diabetes?

20. Do you or does anyone in your family (parents, brothers, sisters) have kidney problems or kidney disease?

Questions 1 to 6 focus on how your weight affects your health overall. Although this information focuses on the "big" problems of health, it also reflects many of the "little" health problems you might have, such as back pain, swollen feet and ankles, knee and hip pain, arthritis, difficulty walking up or down steps, lack of energy, and feeling worn out at the end of the day. The more you weigh, the more likely you are to have health concerns of any kind.

Questions 7 to 15 focus on how your weight affects health problems related to heart disease. Your chances of getting any form of heart disease go up when your blood pressure and blood cholesterol levels go up. You are also more likely to get heart disease if other members of your family have or had heart disease relatively early in life.

Questions 16 to 18 focus on diabetes, which is a health problem in itself as well as a factor in other health problems such as heart disease and kidney disease. Having other family members with diabetes (type 2) makes it somewhat more likely that you will develop this condition as well, although your weight and level of physical activity are the most significant factors.

Questions 19 and 20 concern kidney problems. They are almost always the result of other health problems. Diabetes and high blood pressure are the leading causes of kidney problems and kidney failure. When you have both diabetes and high blood pressure, it is especially important for your doctor to monitor your kidney functions.

What matters more than your answers to these 20 questions is what you choose to do about those answers. Hypertension, heart disease, diabetes (type 2), and high cholesterol are health problems that can affect anyone, regardless of weight. *But when your body is carrying half again to twice as much weight as is healthy, these health conditions are likely to be yours.* Your Menu for Life can change your health status for the better, so you can feel better . . . and feel better about yourself. Alquietta, Cedric, Clarence, Marie, Stephanie, Howard, and many other people who followed the Menu for Life approach through the Obesity Study are living, healthy proof that *you too* can do this!

FACING THE NUMBERS

Did you have trouble answering many of the 20 health questions? When was the last time you went to the doctor? If you can't remember or it has been more than a year, it is time to go. When you weigh too much, you tend to avoid the doctor unless you absolutely have to, until your health problems are so big you can no longer ignore them. Then, if you do go, you say you are there because your loved ones say you snore, because your knee hurts, because the cut on your foot fails to heal—not because you weigh too much!

But the number on the scale *is the reason* you are at the doctor's office, no matter what you *think* is the reason. You do not want to face the scale. Whatever that number is, who needs to know it? Some people's bodies may be so big they are literally off the scale—people have trouble fitting on the scale, or need to be weighed on a special scale. You might try to make a joke out of it (whether you feel like laughing inside is debatable), or you may respond with defiance. This is an act to cover up the truth: the number on the scale startles and dismays you. *So what?* So what do you *do* about it? What *can* you do?

The number of pounds you weigh connects to more startling, unpleasant numbers—the numbers that measure your blood pressure, your blood cholesterol, your blood sugar (glucose). Confronting the numbers head-on, facing them for what they are and what they mean for your health, is the only way to jolt your mind free of letting you believe that fat is fit. When your blood pressure is high, your blood cholesterol is high, your blood sugar is high—*you are not healthy.* When your body weighs too much, your health pays the price.

If you walk into my office and you weigh too much, I know this is why you are here. I know this for two reasons. One is that your weight is a vital sign. Vital signs are the basic indicators doctors use to assess the general status of your health. When I see that you weigh 200, 250, 300, 350 or more, this vital sign tells me your body is suffering under the burden of extra weight it carries as surely as a fever tells me you are fighting an infection. I know all of the changes that take place within your body when you weigh too much, and I know what kinds of health problems these changes cause.

The second reason is that I know the burden of your extra weight causes the problems that bring you to the doctor. You come in because you snore. I want to talk to you about your weight because I know that when you lie down at night to sleep, all that extra body fat presses against your upper body and your throat and makes it harder for you to breathe. You probably have sleep apnea. You come in because your knee hurts. I want to talk to you about your weight because I know your body weighs more than your knees can support. You probably have osteoarthritis, and your hips and your ankles likely hurt too. You come in because the cut on your foot keeps you from wearing your favorite shoes. I want to talk to you about your weight because I know you are likely to have diabetes (type 2), one sign of which is a wound that doesn't heal. And I want to talk to you about your weight because I know you might also have high blood pressure, high blood cholesterol, and any number of other health problems that are common when you weigh too much. I want to talk to you about your weight *because* you weigh too much, and *that itself is a health problem.*

You may struggle with the concept that your health problems relate to your weight. Your doctor might humor your illusions about your weight, indulge your rationalizations, choose to focus on treating the reasons you think you are in the office rather than confronting obesity as a contributing risk factor to serious health problems, as a serious health problem in and of itself. Unfortunately, some doctors are too slow to urge you to stop gaining weight, to urge you to make the changes in what you eat and how you move that will improve your health. If so, *find another doctor who takes your weight problem seriously and wants to help you.* Denying reality does you harm. You might not like what your doctor says about your weight and your health when he or she confronts you about it. That's okay. Some messages are unpleasant to hear. But when your doctor presents you with the truth, these messages give you the opportunity to *change your situation for the better.*

Whatever the numbers are, they can help you because they tell you where you are. As you move toward health, you watch your numbers move toward health—the numbers on the scale, the numbers on the lab reports, the numbers on the blood pressure dial. These are serious numbers, and if you take them seriously you can change them. If you choose to ignore the numbers and pretend they don't matter, soon enough they *won't* matter because you will be too sick to reverse the disease process and return to health and well-being! Listen to what Cedric said and take charge *before* you have a health crisis. Make a pre-emptive doctor's appointment; your doctor's office is where you can, and should, face the reality of your health situation. Step on the scale, *look* at the number. *Remember* the number. Because once you start losing weight, every number that is lower than the number where you started is good! Every time any of the numbers for your blood pressure, your cholesterol, or your blood sugar goes down from their too high levels toward healthy levels, your health improves.

Use this chart to keep track of your numbers.

Date	Weight	BMI	Waist	Blood Pressure	Blood Cholesterol	Blood Sugar

A CONSTELLATION OF HEALTH CONDITIONS

We conducted our Obesity Study because we wanted to find ways to help Americans, particularly African Americans, reduce their risk for cardiovascular disease by lowering their risk for diabetes, hypertension, and hyperlipidemia. Although cardiovascular disease knows no ethnic or racial boundaries, when you are African American you are at especially high risk for the conditions that lead to it for reasons researchers don't entirely understand. As an African American your risk for heart disease is already statistically greater, and when you are also overweight or obese, your risk for heart disease, and for other serious health conditions, compounds and increases further still. Here is what we know:

- Two in five African Americans have some form of cardiovascular disease.
- African-American women now have a higher death rate from heart disease than do white men, who have traditionally had the highest heart-disease death rates.
- An African American between the ages of 35 and 54, the prime of life, is twice as likely as a person of any other ethnicity to have high blood pressure.
- Nearly one in two African Americans has high blood cholesterol; one in six has very high blood cholesterol.
- Diabetes accounts for 43 percent of all kidney failure in African Americans, four times the rate at which it accounts for kidney failure in white Americans. Hypertension accounts for 42 percent of all kidney failure in African Americans.
- Twice as many African Americans have diabetes (type 2) as do others in the general population.

Each of these health conditions—high blood pressure, high blood cholesterol, diabetes—is potentially life threatening. All three conditions are key factors in heart disease. When you have them in combination, they intersect with and compound each other in ways that create other health problems. Look back at the entry data in Chapter 3 that we gave for participants in the Obesity Study who entered the Menu for Life program with one or more of these three health problems. When all these health problems take over, your health status reaches a point where it becomes nearly impossible for doctors to separate one problem from another or to reverse all the damage these health problems have caused. But *when you catch the problems early*, before they become entrenched, before they irreversibly change your body, *you can head off disastrous consequences.* Eliminate the cause of these problems—weighing too much—*before there is damage to your body.*

High Blood Pressure (Hypertension) "When you are nowhere near your 'ideal' body weight, when you are obese and carrying all that weight, you are carrying all kinds of health problems," Stephanie Dove says. "When I weighed 140, I didn't have high blood pressure. I didn't have chest pain. When my weight went up, I got high blood pressure. I had to take medication. I had a cardiac event that put me in the hospital intensive care unit for a week. When I get old I don't want to spend all my time in the doctor's office. I want to live, I don't want to die. And overeating kills you. Being inactive kills you. I don't want to take all these medications that have side effects, all of that. *I want to live.*"

Blood pressure is the measurement of how much force it takes for your heart to pump blood through your arteries. The more of you to pump through, and to, the more you weigh, the more body mass you have, the harder your heart must pump. Doctors write your blood pressure as one number over another: for example, 120/70. The top number, your systolic pressure, is the force your arteries experience when your heart contracts (the beat you feel with your pulse). The bottom number, your diastolic pressure, is the force your arteries experience when your heart relaxes (the space between the beats of your pulse). Both numbers are important.

BLOOD PRESSURE RANGES

Your Blood Pressure Is . . .	If Your Systolic Reading Is . . . (mm/Hg)	and Your Diastolic Reading Is . . . (mm/Hg)
Ideal	less than 130	less than 85
Normal	130-139	85-89
Mildly high	140-159	90-99
High	160-179	100-109
Severely high	180-209	110-119

Many people have high blood pressure and fail to recognize it, because despite the many health problems it can cause, by itself high blood pressure has no symptoms. In most people, hypertension develops slowly, often over decades. The higher your blood pressure, the greater your risk for:

- Stroke
- Heart attack
- Heart problems
- Kidney problems
- Kidney failure

Losing 10 to 20 pounds can drop your blood pressure by 10 points or more, particularly when you make regular physical activity a part of your daily life. During the six months of her participation in our Obesity Study,

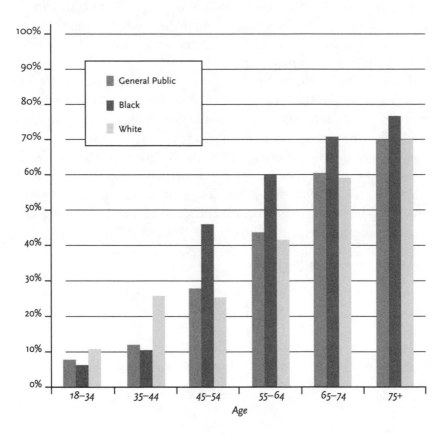

Americans with High Blood Pressure

Stephanie lost 55 pounds. Her blood pressure dropped enough that she could reduce her medication. Excess body weight is not the only cause for high blood pressure, of course. People of healthy weight get hypertension too. But when your weight goes up, so does your blood pressure—and losing weight helps bring it down, even if you must continue to take medication.

How do you know if you have high blood pressure? As we said earlier in the chapter, *you don't unless you have it checked*. Only having a blood pressure reading taken—with a cuff placed around your arm—can tell you whether your blood pressure is high. Most doctors' offices and health clinics and many senior centers offer free blood pressure checks, as do kiosks at shopping malls, drugstores, and grocery stores where machines give blood pressure readings. Get a baseline blood pressure reading from your doctor's office, and then you can use these other resources to monitor your blood pressure as you lose weight and the numbers start to drop. Your doctor will want to monitor your blood pressure too, to make adjustments in your medication.

Diabetes. "I'm from a family with a history of adult onset diabetes," says Clarence White. "I did not want that, and I knew that my weight was putting me on that path. I was already taking medication for hypertension and to lower my cholesterol. I had heard that weight loss and exercise could lower your blood pressure . . . I couldn't believe that, but I knew it must be true. But mostly I wanted to minimize my chances for getting adult onset diabetes. I had two uncles and an aunt who died from complications associated with diabetes, many others on that side of my family who have diabetes. All of them are heavy except one. The more I learned, the more I realized that being overweight is a detriment to your health."

Like any other health problem related to your weight, diabetes (type 2), the kind of diabetes that usually develops in adulthood, does not suddenly appear. In most people it develops over years. As your weight climbs, your doctor might warn you that you have "prediabetes," glucose intolerance, or insulin resistance. All of these terms identify the early stage of imbalance between insulin and glucose (sugar) in your body that, if allowed to progress, will become diabetes (type 2). This stage is your opportunity to keep diabetes from developing.

Your risk for diabetes (type 2) is tied directly to your weight. Excess body fat interferes with your body's ability to use insulin. The more you weigh, the more likely it is that you have diabetes. The symptoms of diabetes (type 2) include:

• Rapid and sudden weight loss
• Increased thirst and urination
• Increased appetite
• Decreased energy
• Vision problems (blurred vision, frequent changes in eyeglass prescription)
• Tingling sensations in your hands and feet
• Skin sores, skin infections, and yeast infections

If you have any of these symptoms, see your doctor for a checkup. A simple blood test can let you know whether you have diabetes (type 2).

It is easy to fool yourself into believing that having diabetes is really nothing to worry about. After all, advances in medications and treatment approaches make it possible to enjoy a relatively normal life when you have diabetes. This does not mean, however, that this disease is kind to your body. The reality is quite the opposite. While you may be going through the activities of your life completely unaware that you have diabetes, diabetes makes a mess out of your body. It is the leading cause of blindness and kidney failure in the United States, and a key cause of heart disease.

When you have *both* diabetes and hypertension, as do many African Americans who weigh too much, you very likely have some degree of kidney disease as well. The high blood glucose levels of diabetes and the pounding effect of high blood pressure combine to put incredible stress on the delicate structures within the kidney that filter your blood. Although many organs in your body can absorb substantial damage before their functions become impaired, your kidneys cannot. Once damage occurs, it is irreversible. Medication often can delay the progression of kidney disease to kidney failure, if you catch it early enough. Kidney disease has few signs until it becomes advanced, at which point there is nothing contemporary medicine can do to reverse it. This is yet another reason that regular medical care is so important when you weigh too much, and is crucial when you have diabetes or high blood pressure (or both). At each visit your doctor can monitor your kidney function through lab tests and catch kidney problems before they become irreversible.

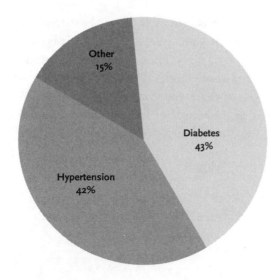

Causes of Kidney Failure in African Americans

Kidney failure is, bluntly, the line between life and death. Without your kidneys, you cannot live. When your kidneys fail, you must rely on dialysis to take over their work—a machine filters and cleans your blood. Black men between the ages of 25 and 44—in what should be the prime of their lives—go on kidney dialysis *18 times more often* than the general population. According to the American Heart Association, hypertension contributes to a *320 percent increase* in end-stage kidney disease among African Americans. Once kidney failure reaches this point, the only permanent solution is kidney transplant. Sound pretty bleak? It is. *Your weight is a health problem.* Getting your weight under control helps you gain control of other aspects of your health.

High Blood Cholesterol (Hyperlipidemia). "As a nurse, I knew about cholesterol," says Alquietta Brown. "I cared for patients who were in the hospital because of the health problems high cholesterol caused, like blocked arteries in the heart and heart attack. But I didn't think much about how cholesterol related to *me*. I didn't connect what I saw every day at work to what could be happening in my own body."

High blood cholesterol is a health problem itself as well as a major risk factor for high blood pressure, coronary artery disease, and heart disease in general. Cholesterol is a fatty substance (lipid) that your body uses for many purposes including to build new cells, repair damage to cells, and transport certain chemicals through your bloodstream (like fat-soluble vitamins, see Chapter 8). Cholesterol exists in your body in several forms. Blood tests measure your blood cholesterol levels. You might hear about good cholesterol, bad cholesterol, cholesterol ratios. But when you weigh too much, you likely have too much cholesterol in your blood. All of these different numbers might be interesting, but what matters most right now is getting your total blood cholesterol down.

BLOOD CHOLESTEROL LEVELS

Cholesterol Level	Healthy (No Health Risk)	Borderline	Health Risk
Total	less than 200	200 to 240	greater than 240
HDL	greater than 45	35 to 45	less than 35
LDL	less than 100	100 to 160	greater than 160
Ratio, Total-to-HDL	less than 3	3 to 4	greater than 4

Many foods contain dietary cholesterol. But for most people, this is not the major source of the cholesterol that creates health problems. Most of the cholesterol in your body does not come from the foods you eat. The cholesterol that creates health problems is the cholesterol that your body manufactures—and a key dietary source for this is saturated fat. Your body continues to make cholesterol as long as it has the sources it needs to do so, and all of the cholesterol your body makes continues to accumulate in your bloodstream. There is no point at which your body says, "enough!" The higher your total cholesterol, the lower your HDL—"good" cholesterol—and the highter your LDL—"bad"cholesterol. We want HDL to be high and LDL to be low. The more HDL your body makes, the better. Limiting saturated fats in your diet limits the source for cholesterol production, which helps to keep LDL down and HDL up. Exercise increases HDL, which further favors a healthy cholesterol ratio.

Insulin plays a role in how your body controls and uses cholesterol. When your insulin balance becomes altered, as when you have insulin-resistant diabetes (type 2), cholesterol has an even greater effect in clogging your arteries. This narrows the passageway for blood, and it takes more pressure now to push blood through your arteries. So your blood pressure goes up. And now, because there's so much cholesterol cluttering your arteries, the intensified surge of blood that comes with each heartbeat carries with it the risk of dislodging fragments of debris. These fragments travel through your bloodstream until they can no longer fit through the blood vessels, at which point they create a blockage. If this blockage is in your brain, you have a stroke. If it is in your heart, you have a heart attack.

Regular exercise is one of the most effective ways to lower your blood cholesterol. All of the changes that take place within your cells, deep inside the inner workings of your body, make your body more efficient at processing fatty acids so they stay in your bloodstream for less time. This gives them less opportunity to collect along your arteries. Sustained physical activity lasting a minimum of 30 minutes (walking your 30 for 5 in Chapter 7) helps your body to use fatty acids as fuel.

Lowering your total blood cholesterol level by just 1 percent reduces your risk of dying by 2 percent. This might not sound like such a big deal, but how happy would you be if every dollar you put in the bank became two dollars? When you lower your blood cholesterol, you get better than a two-for-one return on your investment because of the ways blood cholesterol levels interact with other risk factors for heart disease.

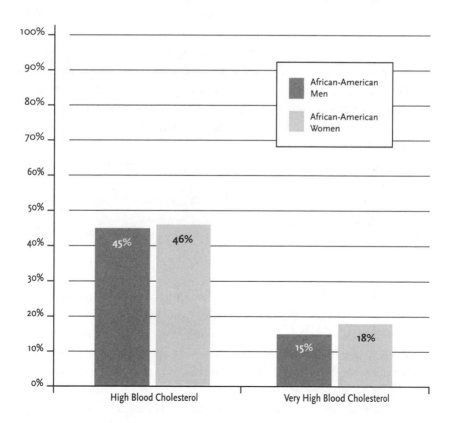

Blood Cholesterol Levels in African Americans

A Menu for Life: Improving Your Total Health Status

Other health problems besides high blood pressure, heart disease, diabetes, and high blood cholesterol can leave you with lasting damage or even threaten your life. When your weight goes up, your risk for certain kinds of cancer—particularly breast, prostate, and colon—goes up too. We don't fully understand these connections yet. What we do know is fat tissue stores hormones such as estrogen (in women) and testosterone (in men), and these hormones affect certain forms of breast cancer (in women) and prostate cancer (in men). With some forms of colon, or colorectal, cancers, it appears that it is the foods you eat that increase your risk. Research continues to explore these connections.

The one connection that seems clear, no matter what the reasons, is this: *Obesity is not a natural state for the human body in health. Obesity is unhealthy.* As long as you weigh too much, your health is at risk. Your weight, by itself, is a health problem, and your weight is causing other health problems. The only way to stop the spiral is to *stop gaining weight.* When we conducted our Obesity Study, we wanted to know how much lifestyle change, in terms of eating habits and exercise, does it take to make a measurable change in health status? The answer: surprisingly little. After just six months, study participants following the same Menu for Life guidelines that we outlined in Chapter 3:

- *lowered their total blood cholesterol 1.4 percent*
- *raised their HDL ("good" cholesterol) 21.4 percent*
- *lowered their LDL ("bad" cholesterol) 10.4 percent*
- *lowered their body weight by 9.1 percent*
- *lowered their BMI by 9.5 percent*

This is exciting news, and we published our findings in the June 2002 issue of the *American Journal of Cardiology.* In addition, the people who went through our Obesity Study experienced many other kinds of health improvements—from decreased dependence on medications to easier breathing and greater range of movement. And you will too when you follow your Menu for Life.

Look around you. Look at family members and friends who weigh too much and have health problems as a result. Remember family members and friends who died young because of these health problems, died young because they weighed too much. Look at the health problems you are developing yourself. "Look around at the elderly," says Stephanie. "You don't see a lot of obese elderly people! Elderly people are thin, because the obese ones die young. Weight adds stress to every part of your body. It makes you look older and feel older than you really are. It gets your joints, your heart. The more you weigh, the closer you are to death!"

The old saying is true: Knowledge is power. Now that you have the knowledge, *what will you do?* Continue on a path of eating too much, making poor food choices, staying inactive, and gaining pounds? Or, will you choose to start your Menu for Life? The consequences of the path from overweight to obesity are clear, and they are dire. There is so much hope in knowing that even a modest weight loss of five pounds makes a measurable, significant positive change in your health status. By acting now you can postpone or maybe prevent a health crisis from occurring. *All by losing weight and keeping it off with your Menu for Life.* Make an appointment to see your doctor. Get moving. Get healthy. Eat well. Lose as much weight as you want to lose. Feel beautiful.

Still unconvinced? Do you want to say, "Dr. Randall, Donna, you don't know what it is like?" Yes, we do. And we know it from both personal and professional experience. "I know the dangers," Donna says. "I've been through most of them. I've had high cholesterol. I have the aches and pains of arthritis. I've had a cardiac event with 90 percent blockage on the back of my heart. *Hello!* Was it the stress eating problems, going from 140 pounds after four kids to 240 pounds? Okay. When you are under stress you may doubt yourself for a while. You do a lot of crazy things when you are under stress. You may have gotten yourself to a place where you are on a vicious merry-go-round where you think you are okay, you are healthy, but you are fooling yourself. If you continue to hide your head in the sand and gain weight, Dr. Randall and I can guarantee you will not like what happens. But you *can* change your health situation. You *must* do so, and you must do so *for yourself*. The change has to come from within you. You don't *need* to be weighed down by health problems. Do your Menu for Life and let your light shine."

6

~~~~~~~~

Energy Out: How a Body Loses Weight

*T*he little things used to be so easy—getting in and out of your car, chasing after your kids or grandkids for a hug and a kiss and *I love you*, or a *Hey, what do you think you are doing now?* (Never mind trying to pick the kids up in your arms and haul them around! Now it's enough to manage balancing a squirmy child on your lap while you sit in a chair.) Reaching, pulling, bending—all the little things you did so easily on days when you found yourself busy, on your feet all the time, going from one thing to the next without sitting down or taking a break. When you give it some thought, you realize the little things aren't so easy anymore, or even always possible.

It takes more energy, more energy than you have, to go through the motion, the movement, of your everyday life. Day by day, year by year, you learn to compensate. You ask someone "taller" to reach up for you, even though height really isn't the issue. You lose your breath walking down stairs, and maybe even your balance once or twice, and then tell yourself, or whoever may be around to hear, that they ought to "fix" that banister! You sit on a chair to reach down, instead of getting down on your hands and knees. Or if you do find yourself sitting or kneeling on the floor, you must pull yourself up to stand again by holding onto something or someone. You lean on the shopping cart in the store, whether you are walking through the aisles or waiting in line for the cashier. Even at work, you turn to coworkers for help with lifting and other physical tasks—and your share of the "help" becomes supervising the action.

You might be able to convince yourself at first that nothing important has changed. You might not even notice you are not moving as much, or as well, as you used to. No matter how old you are, you are not as young as you used to be. You tell yourself people slow down when they get to be adults or when they have health problems. That just makes sense. There are things you can't do anymore, because those are the things younger people, people who are strong and healthy and fit, do. So you stop doing things and do your best to accept that you can't get your body to do everything you want it to do anymore.

Over time you find that all your body wants to do is sit, and no matter where you are or what you are doing, you find ways to accommodate that. Until reading this book, you may not have connected your health problems—like your joint pain or your diabetes—to your weight problem. But now you do; you know that your weight problem is directly related to many of your other health problems. Until reading this book, it may never have occurred to you that avoiding movement and activity *truly* compromises your optimal experience of daily life, your health, and your efforts to lose weight and keep it off. You've told yourself that if you needed to lose weight, you could just diet. You still manage to get things done. How important can moving *be*?

Truth be told, you don't really *feel* much like walking, like getting up and going, because you don't have the energy for it—emotional or physical. Even though you put plenty of Energy In, the left side of the Energy In/Energy Out equation you learned about in Chapter 4, you don't have that energy available to you when your body needs to move. Under the weight of your heavy body, your hips, your ankles, your knees just can't support you well. They aren't as flexible or reliable as they used to be, and putting them in motion takes a lot of effort. Moving much, sometimes moving at all, hurts. Breathing is a chore with even the slightest exertion. You are right in thinking that you stop moving because your body just can't do it anymore. You are wrong in thinking you must accept this state of awkward, heavy discomfort. Your well-being, your health, and your Menu for Life depend upon not only what and how much you eat, but also upon how active, how much in motion, you are.

DONNA RANDALL ⌐⌐

"So many things that happen in life that you have to deal with every day—life is hard sometimes—and the weight problem starts coming. You stop going dancing or doing your favorite sports or playing with the kids, doing the activities that bring you joy, because you are heavy, and tired, and stressed. You find everyone suddenly focusing on your eating. 'He ought not to eat that.' 'Do you know why she is eating that way?'

"No one, I'm telling you, *no one* wants to be so fat that when you wear a pair of pants you wear out the insides of the thighs. You don't want to be so fat that you can't walk up and down stairs. You don't want to be so fat that you need to ask someone else to do everything for you because you can't do things for yourself like you should. When you weigh too much and you find your eating is out of control, that's only half the problem. What you also need to think about, just as important, is *why you stop moving*. You can't let the stress and the weight get you down, depressed, to the point where you stop enjoying moving and engaging yourself in activities you love, with the people you love. You've *got* to join in. As much as you can, put one foot in front of the other. You don't want to stay trapped, weighed down by that heavy body. I *know* what you are feeling. You *can* change your situation. It isn't hopeless. Reach out. Get up. Move off of that couch or chair. You *can*. You *must*. Because moving is *living*."

DR. RANDALL ⌐⌐

"So far we have examined your Energy In, looking at when, how, and what you are eating. You know you need to think about healthy portion sizes, eating less food, and making more nutritious food choices. You know that bringing your weight to a steady state where you are not gaining and can begin to start losing will help you manage or avoid health problems like hypertension, diabetes, and high cholesterol that are connected to how much you weigh. Achieving that steady state balance and then beginning to lose weight, though, means more than just working with your Energy In. You need to work with your Energy Out too. For your new Menu for Life to be successful, you need to eat less food, you need to make better choices about what foods you *do* eat, and you need to *move more*. You need to boost your Energy Out. Both sides of the Energy In/Energy Out equation are *equally* important. You need to work both sides of the equation to get the maximum result."

The human body, *your* body, is designed to move. It may not feel like it right now, but your body *wants* to move. It wants to reach, walk, stretch, twist, bend—even jump and run. Your body functions at its best, inside and out, when it is in motion. But right now, your body weighs too much, and you find the prospect of getting your body moving difficult and daunting. With all the Excess Energy you have stored up as body fat, you'd think it would be simple enough to turn that stored energy into Activity Energy Out. If only you could find a way to do it without lifting a finger!

We admit it is a challenge to get moving after so many years of inactivity. In the beginning, your body is going to resist your efforts to put it in motion. This is to be expected, and this is temporary. Once you get your body moving, get your body into action on a regular basis, you will have a hard time sitting still again. This we promise you. The challenge to get moving is a difficult one, but it is not impossible. *Your body wants to move.* "Now I walk to work and walk home almost every day," says Cedric Williams. "But when I started, when I was big, I hated exercise. You had to drag me out of bed! Then I got into walking, and now I walk everywhere. People always want to give me rides but walking is my exercise. I'll even walk a couple blocks before I catch a bus so I can use that as exercise. You won't see me in a jogging suit or anything like that, but I will get out on the street and walk."

When you are active, your body uses more energy, and you have more energy available to you to use. When you are *inactive*, when your body moves only the bare minimum necessary to get you through your day, you feel sluggish and tired on the outside, and your body is also sluggish on the inside. When Energy In and Energy Out are out of balance, your body functions poorly from the inside out.

LOSING INCHES IS A GREAT FEELING!

Now people do have different body types, and different body types store body fat in different ways, so the way you carry your stored body fat might look very different from the way your neighbor carries hers or your coworker carries his. Fat cells don't pay much attention to where they are located, they accept fat deposits that come to them through your bloodstream in the form of fatty acids. It's like pouring a bucket of fat over your head . . . it sticks where it sticks—from your belly to your butt to your thighs to your fingers and toes. When you gain weight, your body gets bigger everywhere. You accumulate fat deeper inside your body, too, around vital organs like your heart and your liver. When wrapped in fat, these internal organs begin to function less efficiently, and over time this affects your health in negative ways.

When you eat the right foods in the right amounts and boost your body's activity level appropriately, you set the conditions for healthy weight loss. As body fat disappears, the cells that once held the fat collapse. You get thinner, and it shows when you get dressed. Maybe you drop a size or two in your clothing. Losing inches also means you increase your flexibility and range of movement. You can "get out of your own way" when your body is less bulky. Simultaneously, you add strength as your muscles build new tissue to respond to the call for added Activity Energy Out. The end result of this process doesn't show *as much* on the scale, though, because as you remember, fat takes up a lot of space in your body but it *weighs less* than any other body tissue. Muscle weighs more than fat . . . even as it takes up less space.

So, at first, you lose more inches than pounds, which until you understand what is happening inside your body, may seem confusing to you or disappointing. What is happening inside is that you are losing fat, but you are building muscle. The pounds come off more slowly, but you feel and move better, more easily, because you are stronger and more fit. This is something to be proud of. So when people say to you, "Looking good! How much did you lose?" Say, "Two inches around my waist!" When you respond this way, you can rightfully enjoy the positive reinforcement and encouragement you get from friends, family, and coworkers. You know you are doing good things for your health, because as you learned in Chapter 2, there is a direct connection between waist size and risk for heart disease. Losing inches means your body is getting smaller *and healthier*. Feeling better is a more important measure than the numbers on the scale.

When you try to lose weight in just one place, like your waist, success is elusive. Your body simply doesn't function this way, though it may seem like it should. When you start to lose body fat, your face might look thinner before your midsection does. This is because the places where there isn't a lot of room for fat to be stored, like your face, tend to show fat loss sooner, so it gives the illusion that these places lose fat faster. You might notice your wrists or your ankles seem more slender and wonder what's going on with your still-heavy thighs. Don't worry . . . they are losing fat too. It's not as noticeable because there are more fat cells between the skin and the muscles of your thighs and your abdomen than there are in your face.

In our Obesity Study, we had people change their eating habits and their exercise habits all at once. For you, at home, the change in the way you eat and move might take more self-directed effort and patience. And that's okay. Your positive results over time will be the same. People in the study went from eating lots and lots of food that wasn't especially nutritious or good for them to eating less food that was nutrient-dense, but still as flavorful and filling. And they went from sitting on the couch to walking on the treadmill three or four days a week, right away. Because we worked with people in a structured environment, everyone lost weight the first week, and they were very happy. As their bodies settled into the new way of eating and moving, though, people got worried when they didn't seem to lose as much weight as quickly as they did at first. Why weren't the pounds melting away? Meanwhile, their clothes felt too big all of a sudden. You will find, as you do the Menu for Life program, the same thing happens to you. And it is a good thing!

BOOSTING YOUR METABOLISM: HOW YOUR BODY USES ENERGY

We talked about the "black box" of metabolism in Chapter 4, the process through which your body converts Energy In—the food you eat—into one of three forms of Energy Out: Survival Energy, Activity Energy, and stored Excess Energy. Donna and I get a lot of questions from people about having a "slow" or a "fast" metabolism. People ask about this not only in relation to how much they can or can't eat without gaining weight, but also in relation to their energy levels. You hear that people with fast metabolisms use more energy and are more "lively" than people who have slow metabolisms. Just what does this mean? If you have a slow metabolism, how will you lose weight? If you have a fast metabolism, why do you weigh too much? Let's find out.

People do have different rates of metabolism. Your body might use more, or less, Energy Out than does your sister's body, or your brother's body, or your best friend's body. We don't yet know why this is; researchers are doing a lot of promising study on it. However, this truth is universal and scientifically proven: *When you increase the level of your physical activity on a regular basis, your metabolism speeds up.* The more active you are, the more your body moves, the more exercise you get, the faster your metabolism functions.

Whatever energy it takes for your body to stay alive, two-thirds of it goes immediately to support the functions of survival—breathing, circulation, and brain activity. You already know from Chapter 2 that you can't directly change the amount of Survival Energy Out your body uses; internal physiological processes and controls determine what your proper amount of Survival Energy is. But when you increase the overall level of your Activity Energy Out—when you become more active on a consistent basis—your Survival Energy Out picks up to keep up with the new needs of your heart, lungs, and tissues. So even when your body is at rest, it uses more Survival Energy because it is now accustomed to meeting higher Activity Energy Out needs.

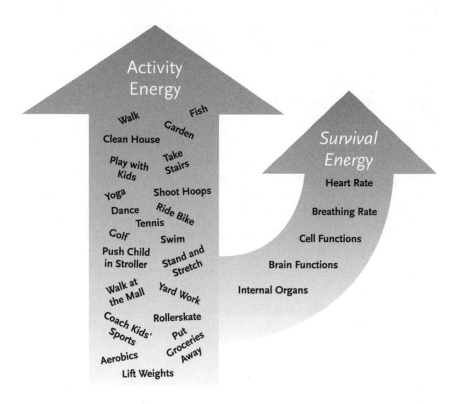

Activity Energy Increases Survival Energy

Your body converts the food you eat, your Energy In, into energy sources available to you for use as Survival and Activity Energy Out—but only as a limited-time offer. If your body doesn't use the energy sources fast enough to meet your Survival Energy Out and your Activity Energy Out needs, your body considers the energy to be good only for storage and converts it to Excess Energy Out: *body fat*. This metabolic process is really a series of cycles, so every stage of the cycle is present in your body nearly all of the time. Each time you eat or drink something, each time you put Energy In into your body, you start a new cycle. All Activity Energy Out draws from these energy supplies, so the more active you are the less extra remains for your body to convert to stored body fat.

The more you move, the more Energy Out your body uses. You move closer to balance between Energy In and Energy Out. When you boost your Energy Out to reach a steady state with your Energy In, there is no Excess Energy to store and pack away. When you boost your Energy Out to *exceed* your Energy In, something amazing happens. You find the metabolic key that unlocks your "storage closet" of Excess Energy. You start *un*packing stored energy . . . just as you might unpack stored clothes from boxes in the back of your closet instead of going shopping for new clothes. Your body turns to what it has been saving . . . body fat, activating it as an energy source.

When you maintain a healthy level of Energy In, between 1,800 and 2,400 calories a day of nutrient-dense food, and boost your Energy Out to exceed that level of caloric value for Energy In, you will lose weight safely and steadily while keeping your body nourished. But when you severely decrease your Energy In, say, on a fad diet, your metabolism shuts down, becomes only minimally functional, and you go into starvation mode. Your energy decreases and your metabolism slows. *Keep eating healthfully!* When you eat at a healthy level and increase your Activity Energy Out appropriately to exceed Energy In, your body keeps giving the signal to boost your metabolism so that you can activate Excess Energy Out and lose weight in a health-producing, vitality-boosting, life-enhancing way.

The food you eat, your Energy In, provides your body with energy from three sources: carbohydrate, protein, and fat. Most of what you eat is carbohydrate, which becomes available as energy for your body within as little as 30 minutes of when you eat it. Carbohydrate is the energy source your body prefers for the functions of Activity Energy Out because it is fast and easy for cells to use. Inside the "black box" of your metabolism, your

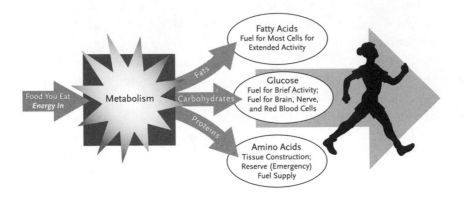

Energy Sources Become Fuels for Survival and Activity Energy Out

body converts carbohydrate energy into the simple forms of sugar, glucose, your cells prefer. Whatever glucose your body cannot use within about six to eight hours, it converts to stored energy. Carbohydrates fuel your body's immediate energy needs, particularly those of activity and exercise. The more active your body is, the more of this carbohydrate fuel source it uses—and the less of it that is available for conversion into stored energy, or body fat.

As you boost your body's activity level, carbohydrates fail to do as good a job of meeting your Activity Energy Out needs. Carbohydrate is an energy source more like a string of firecrackers—your body has to "light" one after another to release energy. This *takes* energy, and your body can do it only for a short time—about 20 minutes. After that, your body needs a more sustained energy source, a steady source to fuel your Activity Energy Out, a source that supplies a reliable, and virtually endless, flow of fuel. Where does your body turn to supplement its fuel supply for Activity Energy Out? To Excess Energy stored as body fat. It takes surprisingly little to put in motion this shift from carbohydrates to fat as an energy source for Activity Energy Out—sustained activity of low to moderate intensity for 20 minutes, such as walking, is enough. For as long as you continue the activity beyond this point, and even for some time after you stop the activity, your body meets its energy needs by drawing from stored energy.

The more accustomed your body becomes to making this shift, the more efficiently it does so, and even makes changes in the way it functions

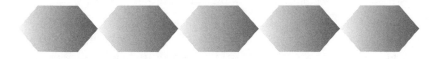

The Release of Energy When Carbohydrate Is the Source

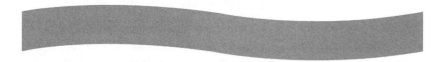

The Release of Energy When Fat Is the Source

to make the process smoother. If you start walking for just 30 to 45 minutes *at one time* five days a week, within about two weeks your body makes three energy-altering adjustments:

• Muscle cells undergo physical changes that allow them to increase the amount of energy from fat that they can use.
• Your heart and lungs develop increased capacity to deliver oxygen to your cells with every breath, which gives your cells the ability to "burn" a higher level of energy from stored fat.
• Your liver lets less sugar (from carbohydrate) into your bloodstream, which causes your body to continue drawing energy from stored fat.

Thirty minutes a day of activity is a very small investment for such major health improvements! What if you can't walk—or engage in some physical activity—for 30 to 45 minutes at a time? Then do it as long as you can! Just by moving, your body becomes healthier. You don't have to move fast and you don't have to move far. You just have to move *steadily*. Every time you put your body in motion, you do good things for your health . . . and you feel better and more energized.

What about protein? How does your body use this energy source? Proteins become amino acids, the substances your body uses to repair and build new cells and tissues including all that muscle mass you build from the new activity you are doing. Some amino acids also serve as an *emergency* fuel supply, because your body can break them down into components that include glucose—the body's fast fuel and the only fuel your brain, nerves, and red blood cells can use. But amino acids are *not* stored Excess Energy. Your body will only turn to protein as an emergency energy source when there is no carbohydrate available to produce glucose.

"In the beginning, you don't think that much about food as energy," says Alquietta Brown. "But once you get started with the regular activity, the regular exercise, it becomes obvious. The exercise is what really gets your body working. At first I couldn't wait to get *off* the treadmill—I hated it! But then I started feeling better, those pounds started coming off, and I grew to love it. You have to stay with the exercise and keep moving. Otherwise everything else you do is a waste."

During the Obesity Study, we measured the effects that walking on a treadmill for 40 to 60 minutes at a time, three days a week, had on heart rate when people first started exercising. The people in the study, people just like you, didn't have much physical activity in their daily lives at that time. Some of them couldn't walk for 40 minutes. They had to stop to rest or walk for a shorter time at first. But it didn't take long for everyone to improve enough to walk at a moderate pace for the full amount of time. After 40 minutes of walking the treadmill, we measured each person's heart rate after 2 minutes, 4 minutes, 6 minutes, and 8 minutes. Doctors have known for some time that the longer it takes the heart to return to its resting rate after exercise, the higher the risk of dying from heart attack. After just three months in the program, we found that people achieve the same peak heart rate while walking, but that their heart recovery rate, the speed at which the heart beat comes back to rest after exercise, improved by more than 10 percent—enough to reduce their risk of dying from heart attack to normal.

What do we learn from this? When you boost your activity level, you can do more and it will cost you less. Your heart is healthier and you have more energy for living. So, very early on in the Menu for Life weight-loss process, within three months, you lose inches and gain health simply by appropriately boosting your Activity Energy. Once you combine this with healthful food portions and choices for your Energy In, you are living your Menu for Life.

Many other changes take place in your body from the inside out when you get regular physical activity, improvements to your health, benefits that increase as you also lose weight. Some of them are:

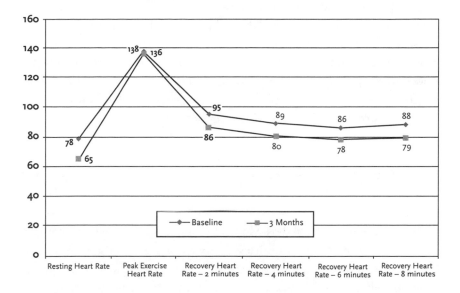

Changes in the Heart Recovery Rate with Regular Physical Activity
Findings from Dr. Randall's Obesity Study

- Your cells become more sensitive to insulin, so they become more effi-cient in how they use glucose (sugar). This is why exercise can improve diabetes (type 2), reducing the need for medication or insulin.
- Your blood pressure drops. As your heart becomes more efficient, it doesn't have to work as hard to send blood through your body. Each heartbeat is stronger, sending more blood at a time. Regular exercise improves the way the cells in your arteries function too.
- Your bones become stronger. Regular physical activity, particularly weight-bearing activities such as walking, helps your bones hold onto the calcium that keeps them sturdy and solid.
- Your immune system is boosted, increasing your resistance to a variety of health conditions from viruses and colds to certain forms of cancer.

The hundreds of people who participated in the Obesity Study experi-enced numerous health benefits, from relief of discomfort from arthritis to blood pressure and blood sugar levels that dropped low enough that they no longer needed medication to control these conditions. Most of these benefits became apparent within a few weeks of beginning to exercise, and as people lost weight their health improvements increased. "When I started taking medication for hypertension, my blood pressure was about 140 over 95," says Clarence White. "I started the Obesity Study on a Monday and I was taking two medications for high blood pressure. On Thursday Dr. Randall took me off them because my blood pressure was too low. I lost 35 pounds when I was doing the program. Now I walk one hour on the treadmill at a gym five days a week, and my blood pressure runs around 124 over 82. Even my asthma is better!"

How Much *Do* You Move?
Your Daily Activity Profile

How active is *your* typical day? Many of us move less than we think we do. And we have more opportunities to increase activity than we realize. Often, your job or other responsibilities dictate the ways in which you move through the work day. But on your time off, or if you are at home with the kids or retired, there are many ways you can boost your Energy Out through increasing your physical activity. Just as with your eating, you need to know where you are, how much physical activity is in your life *right now*, so you know where you can comfortably start to make changes and improvements. Wherever you are right now is the best place to start!

1. How does your body feel when you wake up in the morning and how much effort does it take to get moving?
    _____ Relaxed, rested, and ready for another new day. I get up right away.
    _____ I have a few little aches and pains, but nothing major that keeps me from getting up when I need to.
    _____ I don't mind getting up, but most days I'll lie in bed for a few minutes to let my body "wake up" before I move very much.
    _____ I don't enjoy getting up. My joints ache and often my muscles are stiff and sore. I wish I could stay in bed all day!
2. If you spend most of your waking hours **at work**, what do you do (choose all that apply to you)?
    _____ Sit at a table, counter, desk, or other fixed location
    _____ Stand at a fixed location

_____ Some sitting, some standing
_____ A lot of bending, lifting, and reaching
_____ Walk up and down stairs frequently
_____ Walk indoors
_____ Walk outdoors
_____ Operate light machinery
_____ Operate heavy machinery
_____ Use hand tools or equipment

3. If you spend most of your waking hours **at school**, what do you do (choose all that apply to you)?
    _____ Attend classes all day in the same classroom, with occasional breaks
    _____ Attend classes throughout the day in different rooms, walking within the same building
    _____ Attend classes in different buildings: I ___ walk ___ drive to get around campus
    _____ Mostly sit when I'm in class
    _____ Mostly participate in hands-on activities when I'm in class

4. If you spend most of your waking hours **at home**, what do you do (choose all that apply to you)?
    _____ Care for my own children under the age of six
    _____ Care for other children under the age of six (including my own)
    _____ Cleaning, housework, yard work, shopping, or errands that take at least four hours every day
    _____ Cleaning, housework, yard work, shopping, or errands that take less than four hours every day
    _____ Cook dinner every day
    _____ Favorite hobbies (such as sewing, quilting, knitting, needlework, woodworking, model-building)
    _____ Watch television

5. If you spend most of your weekend waking hours **out and about**, what do you do (choose all that apply to you)?
    _____ Meet friends for breakfast or lunch
    _____ Go to a shopping mall to shop or walk around
    _____ Stay home and sleep to catch up on rest
    _____ Watch television or videos

_____ Meet friends to play cards, cribbage, chess, checkers, or similar activities

_____ Play golf or go fishing

_____ Plan the next week's meals and cook all day

_____ Go boating, sailing, camping, hiking, biking, dancing, or otherwise spend the day outdoors when weather permits

_____ Go see a movie

6. Can you find a style of shoes to wear that is comfortable and allows you to walk?

_____ Sneakers, oxfords, or other shoes with laces

_____ Slip-on, flat shoes that have a complete heel enclosure

_____ Slip-on, flat shoes open in the heel, such as clogs or sandals

_____ I can't find any comfortable shoes for walking

7. When you bend forward at the waist and reach for your toes, what is the lowest body part that you can touch?

_____ Thighs

_____ Knees

_____ Calves

_____ Ankles

_____ Tops of feet

_____ Toes

8. Have you stopped doing a favorite activity that you shared with others? If so, what was it, and what was the reason you gave to the others for stopping the activity?

_____

_____

_____

_____

_____

9. When you were at your most physically active, what activity (not necessarily a sport) did you enjoy the most? What did you love about doing this activity? Do you still do this activity? If not, when and why did you stop? If you could, would you do this activity again now, and how would you go about doing the activity?

_____

_____

_____
_____
_____
_____

10. How often do you turn down invitations to do something because
it involves too much walking or other physical activity?

_____ Most of the time I'll stay home and tell people I've got
other plans or come up with some other excuse why I
can't make it.

_____ I may stay home, but I'll invite everyone to come over to
my house after they're finished whatever it is they are
doing to watch a movie or eat something.

_____ Sometimes I'll stay home, mostly when I'm having a
particularly achy or "bad" day—I just don't feel like going
out and doing things on those days.

_____ I'll go if I know I'll be able to sit down regularly and
then I'll watch the other people do things—I enjoy seeing
people, but I don't enjoy running around all the time.

_____ I go out whenever people ask me to do something and
participate as much as I can in whatever activity they're
doing—as much as I love being social, I love being active
too.

BOOSTING YOUR ACTIVITY ENERGY OUT

"I bought a treadmill when I decided I needed and wanted to lose weight,"
says Marie Primas-Bradshaw. "But even as motivated as I was, I found it
challenging to make sure that I got *on* the treadmill. The exercise part is
the weakest link for me, even though I know how important it is. The
treadmill is right there at home, and I have no excuses for not using it.
Although the treadmill is the answer for me it might not be for you. You
have to find what you like and *do it*. Exercise can be a lot easier too, when
you've got a buddy to do it with. I like taking day trips with friends and
walking on the beach or seeing the sights, wherever we happen to be."

There are dozens, maybe hundreds, of ways for you to boost your Activity Energy Out just doing the regular activities of your life. *Anything* you
do that is more than you do now is a step in the right direction. Sitting

uses more energy than lying down. Standing uses more energy than sitting. And moving—stretching, walking, even just shifting from one foot to the other—uses more energy than standing still. Right now, your bigger body keeps you from moving as much as you should, as much as you want to. Once you start moving, your body starts changing. You feel like moving more, and you can!

Start by identifying all those ways that you compromise on moving your body. For one whole day, sunrise to sunset, write them down in a notebook that you carry with you, to see how many times you decide, sometimes without even thinking much about it, to avoid moving or doing something. Decide not to compromise anymore. Little by little, get yourself in motion and do as much as you can. Start small, don't *overdo* it! If walking rubs your thighs, focus on ways you can move your arms and legs more and do some seated activities until you lose enough inches to walk more comfortably.

Most important, return to doing those things that bring you joy! What would you *like to do*, right now? What is keeping you from doing it? How far could you get if you started out to do it? Getting your body in motion is all about looking at what you *can* do, and then doing it. There are opportunities in every room of your house, every part of your life, to boost your Activity Out.

Your Kitchen. When you bring your groceries home from the store, unload them from the bags onto the counter and then lift them into the cupboard, one item at a time. Give those cans an extra heft or two, like you are working out with weights. Regular cans weigh 14 to 16 ounces—almost a pound. As Donna likes to say, why pay money to join a fitness program that will have you lifting one-pound weights to tone and strengthen the muscles in your arms and hands when you can do the same thing right in your kitchen for no more than you've already spent on groceries! The stretching and reaching to put items away helps you improve flexibility and range of motion too.

Consider rearranging your kitchen so that some things are in lower cupboards, where you bend down to put them away, and others are in upper cupboards, where you reach and stretch to put them away. Remember too: that there is a lot of physical activity in cooking nutritious meals for your family. Really get into your cooking—chop vegetables, knead dough, lift soup pots, check on that roasting pan in the oven. Do as much of the cooking preparation as you can by hand, without the aid of kitchen appliances. Walk around your kitchen when you are preparing meals. Wash and dry dishes by hand and put everything away after your meal is finished. Plates going from dishwasher to table and back to dishwasher again without ever seeing the cupboard is, well . . . we don't need to tell you how we feel about that, you can guess all on your own. And forget about eating straight from the bag, box, or can! You can do better than that, and you'll set a better example for your kids.

Your Living Room. Ah, there it is . . . your favorite recliner, chair, corner of the couch, the spot where you sit when you are home, where you rest and relax. You placed this beloved piece of furniture just so, most likely so it aligns with the television. You probably have a table nearby, so whatever you might want while you are sitting in your comfortable place is within easy reach—the remote control, the television listings, the lamp, a coaster for your soft drink, a place for your snacks. What's wrong with this set-up? *You hardly have to move at all to do anything.* We can remedy that! Start by getting rid of the coasters and the space you reserve on the end table for food. Eat in the kitchen or dining room. This keeps you aware and in control of what, when, and how much you eat. If you want a snack, get up, go to the kitchen, fix yourself some nutritious food, and sit at the kitchen table to eat it. Separate your food from your television set. (And no cheating by putting a TV on the kitchen counter!) Eat dinner together at the table every evening as a family. Yes, we're old-fashioned!

How much *do* you watch television? Watching TV is one of the most inactive "activities" of our modern living. The average American watches more than three hours of television a day. Over a typical lifetime, this adds up to *nine years* by the time you are 75 years old. Think of all you could *do* with nine extra years in your life! Maybe go back to school, spend more time participating in raising your kids, write a novel, learn to cook new foods, dance, sing, travel the world, enjoy living beautifully! When you *are* watching television—and we know you *will* watch it sometimes, watch only what you purposefully want to watch, such as a special news program, sports event, favorite show or movie. Check your *TV Guide* ahead of time. Stand and stretch frequently; do chores or errands around the house not just during commercials but during the show. Nobody says you have to sit still to enjoy a television program.

You might say you watch TV because it relaxes you . . . and it does; you can't be much more relaxed and still awake than when you stare at TV. Even your brain activity slows down when you watch television. You might enjoy lounging in your favorite recliner, with your head back and your feet up, but as far as your body is concerned, you might as well be lying in bed. That's a good selling point for the chair, perhaps, but not so good for your health! Keep the chair in its upright position or switch to a chair that won't let you recline. It takes more energy to sit up than it does to lie down. Move the remote to where you at least have to bend, stretch, and reach to get it. Better yet, walk to the television to change the channel. And even better, turn it off and keep walking! Get outdoors if the weather permits or take a short walk through your house or apartment (if you have steps, walk up and down a few of them as you get stronger).

Same thing with the phone—if you sit and talk on the phone for hours, how much better would it be to get together in person with that acquaintance or loved one and enjoy time doing something together? Many people only have computers at work or at school, but if you have one at home, the same applies there too. Surfing the Internet . . . there's a reason why they call it "cyberspace" and "virtual reality." Hit the escape key and go outside where you can smell the air, feel the breeze on your face, flex your muscles, and know you are walking in the *real* world!

Life is far more interesting face-to-face, experiencing the gift of being alive on this planet with the people we love! Pry your eyes away from the set, hang up the phone, unplug, and find something else to do with your time. Avoid using TV as a baby-sitter for your kids—no dinner and a video. Childhood is a precious time of life's first experiences, but how can a child experience living, how can that child learn, grow, and move, by sitting in front of TV? How can *you*?

Your Bedroom. Your bedroom should be comfortable and peaceful, a place that supports restful sleep. Do you have a television in your bedroom? Collapsing on the bed might feel as if it is the perfect way to relax after a long day, but, like lying on the couch, it takes very little energy. If you are in the habit of falling asleep to late-night TV, move the set into another room. Your sleep will be more restful, and you won't spend as much time lying in bed. At the very least, put away the remote so you have to get out of bed to change channels and turn the television off. If you are not really watching the shows anyway, but keep the television on for background noise to help you fall asleep, turn the radio on instead.

Your Yard. If you have a yard, you have endless opportunities to be active, from mowing the grass and trimming trees to planting a garden . . . and walking around to admire the fruits of your labor. Sitting out in your yard when the weather is nice is more active than sitting on your couch in front of the television, because you are more likely to interact with your environment. So go outside and enjoy the yard. Take time to play physical, outdoor games with your kids. Groom the dog. Wash the car. Or have friends over to play horseshoes or croquet, toss a Frisbee around, walk through the yard with you, even sit outside and play cards, board games, or charades, or just talk. If you don't have a yard, you can cultivate a window box garden or an indoor garden of potted plants—grow your own herbs to use as seasonings when you cook.

Your Neighborhood. When was the last time you went for a walk down the street or around the block? When you got out and about to meet some of the people who live nearby? Maybe you work shifts, have kids to get ready for or pick up from school, or for other reasons you find it hard to go out and take time away from home during the day. A quick walk near your home can let you get outside for some fresh air, to stretch your legs and get your body moving. Maybe your children, grandchildren, significant other, or a neighbor might want to walk with you. Walk the dog, if you have one, instead of letting it out to run unaccompanied in the yard. How far you go and who goes with you, whether human or canine companion, don't worry about it. Go! Have fun, enjoy yourself. Enjoy your companion. Revel in feeling your body in motion and doing as much as you can.

YOUR MENU FOR LIFE: BALANCING ENERGY OUT

Weight loss does not happen *to* you, it happens *within* you. You lose weight when you change the way your body uses energy on the *inside*, and this changes the way you look on the outside. It also changes the way you *feel*, inside and out. Doing your Menu for Life means managing Energy In through the kind and amount of food you eat, as well as boosting your Energy Out by moving more, by enjoying life's activities. If you do both sides of the Energy In/Energy Out equation, you'll feel beautiful, energetic, vital. You'll feel this way after losing only a few pounds, after only a few months of eating better and moving more. You can continue to keep the equation balanced toward healthy weight loss for as long as you want, to lose as much as you *want* to lose, until you reach the place where you are satisfied.

But to be successful, you *must* move. Donna says, "When you tell yourself you *can't* exercise, when you tell yourself you *can't* get out there and dance or walk or do whatever it is that you enjoy, you are wrong. All those *can'ts* again, creeping up on you! What you are saying when you say, *I can't*, is that you can live without your muscles! You tell yourself, 'oh, it's okay to give up my flexibility. I don't *need* flexibility for living. I don't *need* strength.' But honey, you *do* need your muscles and your flexibility and your strength. Activate your Menu for Life and em*power* yourself with the synergy of healthful Energy In *and* Energy Out."

Part Three

~~~~~~

The Program:
Your Menu
for Life

7

~~~~~~~~

Energy Out:
Movement and Activity

*T*hrough the years, Donna and I have heard all the reasons, explanations, and excuses people have for not exercising: "I don't have time." "Exercise is too much work." "I need to lose weight before I can exercise." "I don't have anything to wear." "My whole family is big." "I have health problems." "I don't like to sweat." "I don't want too much muscle." "Exercise is boring." "I can't find anything to do that I like." "I'm too old to exercise; exercise is for young people." And Donna's personal favorite: "Diets make me too weak to exercise!" Whew. That's a lot of complaining and excuses.

Exercise, though, is a very simple thing—perhaps easier than you realize. Exercise is simply a four letter word, and it is a *good* one: MOVE. How do we know when someone is alive? When we see they are breathing and moving! To move is to live. To move is to improve the health of your body, your heart, your lungs, and your mind. Already, you are looking for ways to turn compromises into opportunities for moving. You walk upstairs to get your shoes instead of asking someone else to do it for you. You fold the laundry while you watch your favorite TV show. (You vow never to sit inactive and stare passively at the TV again. And no food in front of the TV either!) You are tending to the yard work yourself, even though it takes you longer than maybe you think it should; it feels good to be outside and watch your efforts take root and blossom.

Once you are moving more and starting to drop a few pounds, your aches and pains begin to subside a bit. You start to notice and enjoy how it feels to swing your arms, to stretch your legs, and lengthen your stride if ever so slightly. You observe how it feels to walk, how your foot feels when it makes firm and purposeful contact with the ground and then pulls back to move you forward. Your body is still big, but it doesn't feel quite as heavy, as awkward, as resistant. As you do the Menu for Life program and shift your Energy In/Energy Out balance toward healthful weight loss and increased activity, your body changes in response.

From the inside out, cell by cell, your body reshapes itself. You do not see these changes early on as dramatic numbers of pounds. That comes over time. Quickly, though, you discover the beneficial changes when you look in the mirror and see the inches you've lost, when you can button or zip your clothes with ease, or you drop to a smaller size. You recognize the change when you wake up in the morning with more energy and you *feel* that get up and go! It feels good. *You feel good* . . . and your body wants (and needs) to move even more. After a while your doctor may tell you that you can take fewer medications. You are healthier. All this happens within a few months of doing the Menu for Life program. You tell people you feel like yourself again. And you mean it.

DONNA RANDALL

"Do you want to know what happens when you really get into doing regular sustained exercise? You learn to like the way it feels, the way *you* feel. You learn to like yourself. Your extra energy and vivaciousness become attractive to everyone around you—your family, your friends, your colleagues. Everyone wants to have that new glow that you have, everyone wants to do what *you* are doing.

"Do you think exercise is too much for you? Too much time, too much effort, too much additional stress on your day? Well, how many minutes are there in a day? Twenty-four hours multiplied by 60 minutes is 1,440 minutes in a day. Multiplied by seven days, that's 10,080 minutes in a week. All you need to do to get your weekly exercise in is to walk continuously for 30 minutes, five days a week. How many minutes total per week do you think that is? One hundred fifty minutes. *One hundred fifty minutes.* Dr. Randall and I are asking you to find 150 minutes out of 10,080 in a week. Now really, how hard is that? How stressful is that?

"Find those 150 minutes every week and they will change your life! Skeptical? *Try it.* Stick with walking 30 minutes five days a week for three months and you'll experience dramatic health benefits. You'll look better, you'll feel better, and you'll be healthier too. Everyone will want to know your secret! Say to those people, 'Hey, come out on a walk with me, and I'll tell you *all* about it.' Get them into walking too and make them your walking buddies; start your own Menu for Life Walking Club. Show and tell is a great way to learn!"

DR. RANDALL

"People, when they start the Menu for Life program, have to make changes in how much food and the kinds of food that they eat. This alone is a lot to accomplish. Battling with food, with eating too much and eating the wrong foods, has been a lifelong challenge for most of the people Donna and I see, and undoubtedly food is a challenge for you too. Many people want to do just that much, just focus on getting their eating under control, and they resist doing the exercise. Their logic is this—one thing at a time, do the food first. But that's faulty logic.

Healthful eating and doing exercise are not separate, but are intertwined in a synergy of health and well-being that balances Energy In and Energy Out. You want to know what one of the best motivators is for understanding how and why you need to make lifelong changes in the amount and kinds of foods that you eat? That's the moment when exercise hooks you, when you begin to see how your body changes outside and how much better it feels inside and you know that you are *living* the Menu for Life Energy In/Energy Out equation. You find that you want to continue, to have more success. All you can think about now is how to eat better, move better, feel better.

"You realize you are using your passion for food and your passion for living to eat healthfully and move yourself away from obesity. Walk away from obesity, and you walk away from more than just obesity as a health problem. You walk away from the risk of high blood pressure, high cholesterol, heart disease, diabetes, kidney disease, cancer, sleep and snoring problems, joint problems, and arthritis. The path of not moving is a path to an early grave. So walk. Keep walking. Every step affirms your commitment, your determination. Walk the path of health and well-being, your Menu for Life."

Most of us already know that exercise is good for us. We don't need anyone to tell us to exercise. But yet, when it comes to doing it, we avoid exercise. About 60 percent of all Americans fail to get the recommended amount of regular sustained activity. *Why?* Perhaps because you think of exercise as "all work and no play" and "no pain no gain." Maybe you remember physical education or gym class from school. Maybe you played sports or served in the military and you remember calisthenics of the "drop and give me 20!" variety. This level of exercise, this intensity of physical activity, kept you thin, kept your body strong and lean back then. "I weighed 165 pounds when I entered the Army 40-some years ago," says Howard Copeland. "My body was good then. But then I got out, and I didn't keep up the activity, the exercise. Over the years, I got bigger. Other people could see how big I was getting, but I couldn't really see how big I was. I was huffing and puffing all the time, even to tie my shoes."

Like Howard, over the years many people drift away from vigorous exercise to regular exercise to occasional exercise to arrive, ultimately, at no exercise—without realizing the cumulative influence being inactive has on their bodies and on their lives, on what they are able to do. In the real world, maintaining vigorous fitness regimens for years on end seems unappealing to most everyone. Without a drill sergeant, a trophy, or a multimillion dollar contract it is hard to find the incentive to do vigorous levels of sustained exercise year in and year out. As much as we may want to "be like Mike," swing a club like Tiger Woods, or dance across the stage with the athleticism of Janet Jackson or Tina Turner, that kind of performance is elusive for most people. Setting vigorous exercise goals may not be realistic!

Meanwhile, other responsibilities of life rush in to make demands on your time and efforts. Even regular sustained exercise becomes a luxury, and often one that seems self-indulgent. "The hardest part for me—to find the time, to make the time, for exercise," says Marie Primas-Bradshaw. "I joined a health club and loved it, but I didn't want to get in the car and deal with the traffic just to go. I had lots of excuses, but in reality, they often are real reasons. When you have a challenging career and small children at home you have to prepare for your job for the next day *and* help with homework, and there are only so many hours in the day. The challenge is to find time to do what you need to do for *yourself*, and this is something you *must* do."

Maybe too you feel so much pressure and stress in your life you feel unable to deal with exercise. The *woulds*, the *coulds*, and the *shoulds* overtake you, and the whole idea of exercise seems beyond your reach. So instead of exercising to make yourself feel better, you *eat* to make yourself feel better. Stress eating replaces exercise, and the more weight you gain the more impossible the prospect of moving seems. Your big, bulky body *defies* movement. You enter that self-defeating cycle of obesity where stress and emotional eating trigger obesity and obesity triggers more inactivity and more eating.

As you put on pounds it seems easier to lose weight by dieting rather than to do it by exercising. Man or woman, you go from one fad diet to another, but you are never quite satisfied with the results. *Why?* You are not satisfied because when all you do are fad diets, you are not working both sides of the Energy In/Energy Out equation to promote maximum health and achieve optimal results. To succeed for the long term, your efforts to lose weight *must* combine *healthful* changes in eating habits. (This eliminates most fad diets right there, as fad diets ask you to make *un*healthful changes in eating habits.) with *increased physical activity*. "I tried diet after diet, but I didn't stick with any of them because I didn't lose enough weight fast enough and keep it off," Howard says. "But it's not just about the weight. You have to change your food, *and you have to do the exercise*. It's the only way. I lost 30 pounds in three months with the Menu for Life program, and I'm very happy with how I look and feel. I didn't realize how big my belly was until I lost it."

PUTTING EXERCISE TO WORK IN THE ENERGY EQUATION

On the Energy In side of the equation, we look at the energy value of foods. We know, through scientific analysis of a particular food's nutritional composition, how much of each of the three energy sources—carbohydrate, protein, and fat—a specific quantity of that food delivers to your body. Whether you eat slowly or fast, eat early in the morning or late in the evening, eat the food all at once or eat in portions throughout the day, whether you are man or woman, old or young, these values do not change. The energy value of a tomato or an orange is constant for the *same amount* of that food, no matter how you eat it or who you are. On the Energy In side of the equation, we look at eating nutrient-dense foods that target a daily energy value of 1,800, 2,100, or 2,400 calories. This is a level that provides adequate nourishment and energy to your body and is not too much or too little food to fuel your basic Energy In/Energy Out needs. (If your reason for not exercising is Donna's favorite: "Dieting makes me too weak to exercise," then you are getting *in*adequate nutrition to support your daily energy needs.)

The processes of metabolism that determine how much Activity Energy Out your body requires to balance your personal energy equation toward healthful weight loss are complex. Many factors affect your body's Energy Out needs. To tip the balance of your energy equation toward weight loss, your body needs to use enough Activity Energy to burn up the Energy In so that there is no extra energy for your body to store as Excess Energy, or body fat, plus a little bit more. Your body has to use more calories as Energy Out than it is consuming as Energy In. For our Obesity Study, we calculated how much Energy Out that would be, based on Energy In within the target range of 1,800 to 2,400 calories per day. Time after time, person after person, calculation after calculation, we came to the same conclusion for the appropriate level of Energy Out. For virtually everyone, it takes the energy equivalent of walking continuously for 30 minutes five days a week to lose weight at a safe and healthful pace.

Yes, all you have to do is walk 30 for 5 and you will get your exercise. It is as easy as that. As the weight and inches come off because you are eating less (and more nutritious) food and getting daily regular sustained activity, your body becomes stronger, healthier, and more efficient.

You may wonder if you *really* have to walk for 30 minutes continuously. People ask us this all the time. Yes, you do. The key to losing weight and to keeping it off is to maintain regular sustained exercise as your daily fitness routine. Every time you put your body in motion, you improve your health and boost your Energy Out. When you put your body in *sustained* motion, movement over a period of time, you trigger the metabolic process that allows your body to access stored body fat as Energy Out. But this only happens, your body only accesses body fat as Energy Out, when you do regular *sustained* exercise, continuous exercise that lasts at least 30 minutes.

When it takes your breath away to walk for just five minutes, you might not believe you will ever be able to make it through walking for 30 minutes. Start slowly and do as much as you can. Whether you walk on a treadmill at the community center, walk around your living room, or walk around the block, do what you *can* do. Every day, you will be able to do a little more, go a little farther. Before too long, you will achieve the goal of walking for 30 minutes at one stretch without stopping. This in itself is a worthy goal. Celebrate when you reach it! The more you walk, the more you will be able to walk, until you reach your next goal of achieving 30 for 5. "When I first started, it was very hard," Howard says. "You've got to have the will power to stick with it because it works. *It really works.* I think

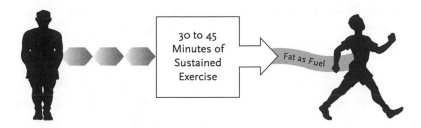

Walking to Use Body Fat as Activity Energy Out

it's the most important and enjoyable thing I've ever done in my 63 years of living."

"When I started to exercise I became more aware of my health status, and my health status was not good," says Stephanie Dove. "For my health, I needed to get the weight off. I *wanted* to get the weight off. I was willing to make the commitment to exercise on a regular basis, to change the way I was eating, because I really wanted to improve my health. When the weight started coming off, what surprised me the most was that I had so much energy!"

READY, SET, WALK!

Walking is the least expensive exercise program you can begin. There are only two things you must do to start: (1) Consult your doctor. (2) Buy a good pair of shoes!

Before you start walking, or doing any kind of exercise, make an appointment to see your doctor. With your doctor, discuss your exercise plans and be ready to have your doctor follow your progress and perhaps do some regular medical tests to monitor any health problems you may have. Exercise benefits nearly all health conditions, as long as you start gradually, work within any limitations that those conditions create for you, and pay attention to the messages that your body sends you. One reason we recommend walking is because it is something nearly everyone, regardless of health conditions, can do and enjoy.

For some health conditions, however, you need to consult with your doctor before making *any* significant changes in your activity level. If you have one of these health conditions, you need to talk with your doctor before you start walking:

- Diabetes for which you take oral medication (pills) or insulin (shots)
- High blood pressure for which you take medication
- Heart problems for which you take medication

These situations are particularly important for a reason that might surprise and will definitely please you. They improve so rapidly and dramatically with exercise that you could suddenly find you are taking *too much* medication. Your doctor can closely monitor your progress and the changes that result in your body as you lose body fat, inches, and weight and adjust your medication(s) to keep pace.

Once your doctor is on board with your fitness goal of walking 30 for 5, go shopping for the right pair of shoes. This is one area where skimping does you a disservice. Invest in good shoes. Shoes that are worn out or run down cannot give your feet, ankles, knees, and hips the support they need. And if you can't support these vital structures, they can't support you! If you have diabetes, which can affect the blood circulation in your feet as well as the healing process for wounds, you need to be especially careful to prevent blisters, cuts, and other problems with your feet. When your feet are comfortable and happy, the rest of you will be more than willing to go where they lead.

A walker all her life, Donna has lots of experience choosing shoes. "No, I'm not a professional shoe salesperson. I'm just a mom who has four very active children who, among them, ran track for nearly 10 years!" Here are Donna's tips for buying shoes:

- Go to a store that has a reputation for knowledgeable sales people and specializes in sports or athletic shoes. Look for cross-training shoes designed for aerobics, running, and walking. These styles typically feature stable yet flexible construction.
- Put on a pair of medium thickness athletic socks. If you don't already have these, buy a pair at the shoe store and wear them to try on shoes. Good socks help to wick away moisture when you walk and to keep your feet dry.
- Have the sales person measure both feet. Try on different brands of shoes, in the size that the fitting device indicates you wear as well as a half size larger and half size smaller. Put on both shoes and walk on a hard surface (not carpet).
- The shoe's heel cup should hold your heel firmly in place, without

allowing any up/down or side-to-side movement when you walk. Make sure the shoe has good padding around the ankle and under the heel, to cushion and protect your foot.

- Leave each pair of shoes on your feet for at least five minutes, unless the fit is clearly wrong. Stand or walk during this time. Does any part of the shoe rub? Pinch? Fit too tightly? Fit too loosely?
- Take the shoe off, hold it at the heel and at the toe and try to bend it. It should flex somewhat, but not feel like it folds up.
- If you can't decide between two pairs of shoes, put the left shoe from one pair on your left foot and the right shoe from the other pair on your right foot. Walk around for five minutes. Choose the shoe style that feels more comfortable.

Expect your feet, and your shoe needs, to change as you become stronger and lose weight. Under the most ideal circumstances, the life expectancy of a pair of walking shoes that you wear five times a week is three to six months. Save your cross-trainer shoes exclusively for your exercise walking or buy two pair—one for everyday use and one for exercise walking. If you use your walking shoes for everyday activities, they will wear differently, making the shoes uncomfortable and less effective when you walk purposefully for your exercise.

Get ready for your walk as though it is a special event . . . because it is. Walking is something you do just for you, an investment in your health and your future. Put on your comfortable clothes and your walking shoes. With all the advancements in sports technology, you can choose walking clothes and socks made from fabrics that wick moisture away from the body and make it easier to move. Depending on how big your thighs are, you might experience chafing when you first start walking. You can minimize this by sprinkling a small amount of baby powder or cornstarch on the surfaces that rub together; do each surface, both legs. Are there other parts of your body that rub, such as your arms, your knees, your calves? Your posture and your body style affect this. You can powder these too.

If you walk outdoors, be sure to dress appropriately for the weather. Layers work best, so as you warm up you can take items off. Choose a route where you can stop and rest frequently at first, if you need to, and where there are not a lot of stairs or a lot of car traffic or stoplights if you can (such as a city park with walking paths and lots of benches, or a suburban nature trail). Walk around your community. Walk with a neighbor, your kids, partner, or friends. Walk the dog. Walk by yourself. Whether you walk indoors or outdoors, keep a bottle of water with you and stay hydrated. You can walk with a pedometer too if you like, a computerized device you program to show you how many steps you've walked and how many calories your body is using. Pedometers can be a fun way to keep track of your progress.

You might want to create your own environment for walking at home, on a treadmill. "I'm not an extreme weather person, so I just never could think of myself being out there when it's raining or whatever," Marie says. "I need something I can do indoors, no matter what the weather is. So I finally bought a treadmill to use at home. I got the one that tells me how many calories I'm burning and how far I'm going. I have it in my office at home where I can have the TV on, or read a magazine if I want. I also have a hands-free telephone, if I want to talk to someone." Walking on a treadmill is a great way to keep the weather, your work schedule, your family obligations, and other "reasons" for not exercising from becoming valid. Walking at home alone can be boring for some people over time though, so you may want to explore walking the treadmill at your local community or fitness center, where you can meet new people, talk, and walk together.

If you are a people person and you like walking with a buddy or a group, you might want to try mall walking. Many shopping malls open early, before the shops open, so people can walk the mall. Some malls and communities have "mall walker" clubs that meet to walk and socialize. It is fun and motivating to share experiences and support with others who are also walking. When you walk with a group, there are likely to be people of all fitness levels participating. Some will be further ahead on the curve than you are, and others will be looking at you with envy and awe for the progress you have made. Expand beyond the mall (or if the mall's not your thing . . .) and plan day trips with your walking buddies to visit museums, gardens, historic homes and landmarks, the zoo, the beach, and other attractions that offer tours or provide good opportunities for interesting walks.

Walking need never be the "same old, same old." Walking is as close as your living room and as far as your feet, your walking buddies, and your imagination will take you. Wherever you walk, choose an environment that is comfortable *for you*. Walking is about real-life fitness, with real-life people. "All those advertisements on TV for gyms, they're a turnoff," says

Cedric Williams. "If they would show people like me, I'd probably be there. But they show these toned people who don't even *need* to be there. I want to be with people *like me*, see and talk to people with *struggles like mine*. Show me somebody that looks like me, somebody who has to *work* to stay in shape. In terms of elasticity, my body's never going to look like that, even when I keep the weight off. My body's not going to be tight. I still have a lot under my shirt, and it's not a six-pack of abs! But I accept that reality. My blood sugar is under control, my blood pressure is under control, I feel better. And although it's not about looks, I do look better too. You don't have to buy equipment or look like a bodybuilder. Just get out there and walk. I walk to work and walk home every day, and I love it."

People say to us, "Okay, this all sounds great, but in *my* life I don't have 30 minutes a day for walking. That 150 minutes a week may not sound like much but it is *a lot* when you have a lot of responsibilities." Donna says right back, "Whether you talk to your mother on the telephone every day, watch television when you get home in the evening, or go for a walk, *the same amount of time goes by*. How are you going to use it?" Just like you, Donna and I have to *choose how to use* the time in our days and when we choose to walk, we find the time without having to look too hard or make a lot of sacrifices about what we are doing. Walking is a natural priority in our lives, something we need and want to do every day!

Donna likes to walk outdoors as much as possible, so she can enjoy fresh air. She walks around local neighborhoods, walks to do errands when she doesn't have a lot of things to carry, and sometimes walks or jogs on a local school track when she really wants to get out and work her body. She walks with our children, who are now adults, when they are available to join her, and with her grandchildren. She walks with her mother or her sister. She walks with friends and with neighbors. She walks with other people that she meets who are also out walking or who want to walk but don't want to do it alone. And occasionally she walks by herself, because sometimes part of the joy of walking is the freedom it gives you to get away from everything else in your life for a little while.

My schedule with research projects and patients keeps me indoors most of the day, so I start my day by parking in an outdoor lot some distance from the hospital building to make sure I get fresh air every day. Like so many hospitals, Howard University Hospital has many long corridors that connect new and old parts of the structure. Although this is less than efficient architecture, it presents endless opportunities for me to walk. Instead of using the phone, I walk to the offices and locations of colleagues when I need to consult with them. I take the stairs instead of the elevator and try to get outside for a walk during the day.

BEYOND WALKING: MOVING YOUR WAY TO MORE NEW ACTIVITIES

As you become more comfortable with the level of physical activity regular sustained exercise brings into your life, look for other activities that you enjoy. Once you reach your goal of achieving 30 minutes of sustained walking five days a week, a state at which your body is strong, flexible, and consistent in its responses, you can vary your experience by choosing to get your exercise in ways other than walking. Many sports and activities get you out with other people as well as keep you moving—and they don't require vigorous intensity to enjoy them. Gardening, golf, shooting hoops, bicycling, running, swimming, water aerobics, dancing, and exercise (aerobic) dance are but a few of the many activities that you can do at varying levels of intensity depending on your ability and interest. The activities of your everyday life can also double as your regular sustained exercise, or they can supplement what you are doing for exercise (depend-

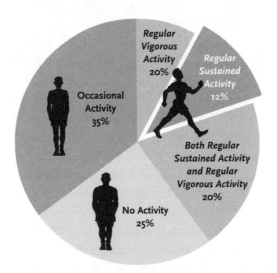

Level of Physical Activity among Americans

ing on how much energy that activity uses). The more you move, the more active you are every day in the things that you do, the more physically fit overall you will be.

To achieve the right level of Activity Energy Out that will allow you to continue losing weight by doing something other than walking (and to keep the weight off), you need to find something you like to do, that you *will* do, and that you can *sustain* for 30 minutes that also requires as much energy as walking does. Here is a list of activities that require more or less energy than walking:

These Activities . . .	Use This Level of Energy Out (Calories) When You Do Them for 30 Minutes
Playing cards or board games, folding clothes, doing laundry, driving a car	60 calories
Putting away groceries, bowling, fishing, playing Frisbee, walking 1 mile	90 calories
Gardening, cleaning house, leisurely riding a bike, walking 1 1/2 miles	120 calories
Dancing, shooting hoops, playing golf, washing or waxing the car, pushing a stroller 1 1/2 miles, raking leaves, water aerobics, walking 1 3/4 miles	150 calories
Mowing the lawn, low-impact aerobics, walking 2 miles	180 calories
Leisurely swimming, exercise dance, riding a bike at 10 mph	210 calories
Playing casual tennis, moderate lap swimming, jogging, riding a stationary bike, walking 2.5 miles	240 calories

If you struggle with exercise and finding ways to get enough exercise, consider this: even athletes find it a challenge to redefine balance in the Energy In/Energy Out equation once they retire from professional sports. When they leave the team, they leave the training. If an athlete ate 6,000 calories a day when competing and continues to eat at that rate after leaving the game, he or she is going to be struggling with weight issues before long. In my conversations with former football great, the legendary linebacker, Deacon Jones, we talked about how hard it is for former athletes to readjust their Energy In to balance with the much lower Energy

Out that they have when they are no longer doing two-a-day drills with games every week.

In his life after pro ball, Deacon Jones *walks* for exercise, he *golfs* for exercise, and he concentrates on eating the right foods in the right amounts. The extraordinary conditioning that was part of his life when he played professional football gave him the ability to function at the high level of a professional athlete only *while he was doing it.* Today, Deacon Jones adjusts his eating and his exercise—like you do—to achieve the healthy steady state balance his body enjoys and that is appropriate for him *now.*

REMEMBER TO BREATHE AND STRETCH

The same aspects of your body's heaviness that make it hard at first to get your body moving also affect your lungs and your breathing capacity. When you start walking and exercising, you need to remember to stretch and breathe. Before beginning exercise you need to warm up. Doing yoga's mountain pose is a great way to warm up. Mountain pose is easy, anyone can do it. Doing this pose prepares you for walking by helping you to center your body, notice your posture and work on your balance. It also helps you open your lungs to take in full, deep breaths. To do yoga mountain pose:

- Stand with your feet as close together as you can without struggling for balance. Shift your weight back and forth and from side to side until you feel you are standing with the same pressure on each leg, and on the heel and toes of each foot, with your weight equally distributed and centered. Leave your arms at your sides, palms facing in toward your body. If standing in mountain pose is uncomfortable for you, do the pose seated in a hard-backed chair with your feet flat on the floor.
- Take a deep breath in, stretch down through your fingertips and up through the top of your head. Feel the mountain rise as you stand straight and tall! Breathe out slowly.
- Breathe in deeply once more, this time lift your heart and drop your shoulders as you press down through your fingertips. Hold for a moment and breathe out slowly.

- Breathe in deeply one more time, press down through your fingertips, lift your heart, drop your shoulders and tighten your buttocks and leg muscles as you feel your foundation of mountain strength build and center itself. Hold for a moment, breathe out slowly, and smile.
- Breathe in deeply, raise your arms over your head, and stretch up. Hold the breath for a moment and exhale, releasing your arms. Laugh. Shake out your arms and legs and start walking!

Yoga helps you become aware of and in tune with your body in many healthful ways, from easing and strengthening your breathing to lowering your blood pressure to increasing your range of movement, and improving your balance. Yoga breathing and meditation exercises are great for stress relief as well as cardiovascular fitness. Even if your flexibility is limited, there are yoga postures you *can* do. A qualified yoga instructor will help you find the right postures for your fitness and health. Most communities have classes in yoga that can be basic and are open to everyone. Yoga is the perfect complement to any other kind of physical activity you are doing.

As you walk and exercise, you may find yourself short of breath because your cardiovascular system is out of shape too, and this can feel a little scary. Shortness of breath catches your attention in a major way, because it keeps you from doing just about anything. As you begin to lose body fat, the pressure that your heart and lungs feel lessens and breathing becomes easier. If breathing during walking or exercise becomes difficult, stop to rest. Stop to rest well before you are unable to catch your breath. If you cannot talk, you are breathing too hard.

When you stop, sit, or stand in yoga mountain pose you open your chest capacity, shoulders down, heart lifted, and head up. This lets your lungs take in as much air as they can, and the pose also helps the rest of your body relax. When you can breathe in a slow, deep, and rhythmic pattern again, return to your walk. Your cardiovascular capacity will rapidly improve as your exercise becomes consistent and also as you begin to loosen the restrictions that your extra body fat places on your lungs and heart.

ACCOMMODATING YOUR HEALTH CONDITIONS DURING EXERCISE

It is normal to feel some soreness when you first start walking or exercising after being inactive for a long time, but *pain is not normal.* You should not experience pain with activity, and if you do, stop right away. Pain is a clear and unmistakable message from your body that something is wrong, and it is a message you must heed. Nearly always, the kinds of injuries you might get from mild to moderate exercise are what we call soft tissue injuries—muscle pulls and mild ligament strains. The best treatment for these injuries is prevention: warming up beforehand, wearing appropriate gear. If they do occur, putting ice on them helps them feel better. Most of the time, it's actually better to gently exercise even when you have a sore muscle or joint. The movement gets blood flowing to the area, which aids your body's healing processes. If your discomfort lasts longer than two weeks, it's a good idea to have your doctor check you out.

Do you have osteoarthritis or other joint problems? Such problems can make some activities difficult for you to do at all or they feel uncomfortable when you do them. Although it seems counter-intuitive, getting your body moving is generally good for these problems. Movement helps to increase your range of motion, flexibility, and strength. If walking or exercising causes you persistent or deep pain, you do need to have your doctor check you out. But if you have simple aches and discomforts, it is likely you will feel better as your exercise becomes more consistent. Do you have problems with your joints, like your hips or knees, or your back? You might find water activities such as water aerobics and casual swimming are easier on these vulnerable areas. Water's buoyancy helps support your weight, which puts less stress on your joints.

When you first begin exercising, we want you to take it easy with the idea of lifting weights or doing any kind of strenuous resistance types of exercise. When your body is big and you weigh too much, the stress created by weight-bearing exercise can cause injuries. You can break a bone or hurt an ankle more easily. Start with walking, light aerobic activities, and yoga, which are safer for you to do and every bit as effective in boosting Activity Energy Out and enhancing your health.

GOING THE DISTANCE WITH YOUR MENU FOR LIFE

"In the Obesity Study, it helped that we were there as a group," says Marie. "We were able to support each other and hear each other's experiences, understand what caused us each to be in our overweight situations. You can do this Menu for Life on your own, of course—it has to be your own, really. But it helps if you can get one buddy, someone to go for walks with, talk to, call, or do this together. You need to have at least one other person who understands what you're going through, to give you support when you struggle and to praise you when you do well."

Listen to people talk when you are shopping, at work, at church . . . you might be surprised to hear how many people in your circle of acquaintances share your desire to move to healthier bodies and lifestyles. Invite some of these people to join you on this journey. A buddy system can be an empowering and fun way to move forward.

When something happens in your life that derails your best intentions to exercise regularly, it is easy and understandable to feel depressed. Setbacks happen for all of us. Sometimes these setbacks seem overwhelming. But there are *always* solutions; some just require more creativity, more innovation, than others. "You take one day at a time and you keep in the forefront of your mind that you've come to this point, a major milestone," says Marie. "It is empowering to remind yourself that you have *accomplished something* and that you *can* maintain your success."

If you are recovering from illness, injury, or surgery, you might have physical limitations that keep you from moving. As your recovery progresses, increase your activity at a rate your doctor advises and your healing accommodates. If the lower part of your body is affected, work your upper body. If your upper body is impaired, do leg lifts, walk or march in place, or stretch your legs and rotate your ankles. Everything you do to keep moving helps your body to stay strong and efficient, to heal . . . and to maintain your Energy Out. Ask your doctor to refer you to a physical therapist who can help you do special exercises to benefit your specific condition and help you boost your exercise safely in general ways as well. When recovering from illness or injury, most insurance companies will cover the services of the physical therapist.

When other problems—family, job, life in general—create stress and challenges, stay tenacious. Find ways to work exercise into your daily schedule and keep it there. In addition to all of the other benefits exercise provides for your body, it also releases chemicals in your brain that elevate your mood and help you feel less depressed. Go to yoga or meditation class. A walk alone might be what you need to get a much-needed break from the source of your stress. Or a walk with friends might provide a welcome diversion from the thoughts and worries that threaten to engulf you. Nearly always, finding ways to make time for exercise, for walking, helps you feel better and think more clearly.

Whether you are facing challenges from illness, injury, stress, or simply because of life's ups and downs, avoid using food to solve your problem. Eating more of the wrong foods is false comfort. If you need to use food for comfort to help you through, focus on reinforcing your efforts to eat healthful foods in the correct portion sizes. Choose fruit instead of candy, lowfat frozen yogurt instead of ice cream, pretzels or crackers instead of chips, cheese instead of high-fat spreads and dips. Eat as much fruit as you want, but put what the package says is a serving size into a bowl so you have to think, and make choices, about how much of other snack foods you are eating. Knowing that you are nourishing your body in the healthiest way possible can help empower your heart and soul and give you the courage to keep walking, one step at a time, one day at a time.

Things happen in life. If you find that you slip toward your old habits of moving less and eating more, do what you did when you first started your Menu for Life. *Start from where you are now.* You know what to do; you've been doing it. There is no day like today, no time like the present to step forward with confidence. Get yourself back to a steady state balance of Energy In and Energy Out, and stay there until you feel comfortable. Use your steady state to ride out the crisis in your life. When things calm down, work again on shifting the balance of your energy equation to weight loss, if that is what you want to do. Your Menu for Life is a process, a journey. Donna tells people, "At first, it might feel that walking a quarter-mile is an almost unbearable distance. But give yourself a chance. It has been a long time since you asked your body to carry you. Be *kind* to yourself. This is not a race, a competition. It is a road, a life-path you are walking—your Menu for Life for the rest of your life. Dr. Randall and I are there with you when the walking is easy, and we are there with you when the going gets tough too. The important thing is to keep walking, keep moving. Participate. Live."

8

~~~~~~~

Energy In:
Diet and Nutrition

*T*hrough the years, Donna and I have heard all the reasons, explanations, and excuses people have for eating poorly. "I'm too tired to cook when I get home." "My wife/daughter/husband/son is the cook and I have to eat what they make." "Learning to cook is too hard and takes too much time." "Cooking meals from scratch with fresh ingredients all the time is too expensive." "My wife/daughter/husband/son eats different things than I do and I end up having to make something different for everyone at each meal—that's too much!" "When I'm on the run I have to get my food wherever it is fast and convenient." "I'm hungry all the time; if I cooked I'd have to live in the kitchen!" "It takes too much effort to eat right all the time—eat this, don't eat that. It is hard enough to stick with a diet for a couple of weeks. It is too exhausting, almost impossible, to consider eating like I'm on a diet for the rest of my life."

We hear people say these words, make these excuses, every day. But we have yet to hear anyone tell us, "I eat fast food because it tastes so good!" Or, "I love eating foods from a box, bag, or can because they give me the best taste and nutrition!" On the menu board or on the wrapper, the food *looks* good and looks like it should taste good. The price is right and everyone in the family can order or ask for whatever they want. Never mind that your meal doesn't look like the picture—or taste like the picture makes you think it will taste—when you unwrap your food in the restaurant or heat it up at home and eyeball what is there on your plate (if you're even using a plate). By that time, you and your family want the food so badly, you put it in your mouth without even thinking about how it *really* looks or tastes, so long as it fills you up and no one is complaining. (Or if they do complain, it's not your fault—everyone got what they wanted.) So why don't you feel better than you do?

Eating healthfully is easier, more enjoyable, and more achievable than you think. Already you are thinking about the Menu for Life Energy In/Energy Out equation and where you are in its balance. You know that if you are getting too much Energy In and you are not moving or exercising, your body will process the food you eat into Excess Energy stored as body fat. You are looking hard at the amounts of food you eat and at the kinds of foods that you are eating. You know you need to eat less food and to carefully consider your portion sizes. You are also considering your eating patterns—from both a logistical and practical perspective (where do you eat and why do you need to eat that way?) and an emotional perspective (why do emotions sometimes make you want to overeat or eat the wrong foods?).

You are also realizing something you knew all along—by and large, fad diets are unhealthful ways to eat and lousy ways to lose weight and keep it off. The only thing that is fun about a fad diet is the glee of watching the pounds come off fast. But the food the fad diets require you to eat and the way you have to eat it is no fun. And it's certainly not fun when the diet is over and the pounds come back again—and then some.

In this chapter, we're going to talk more specifically about the nutritional properties of foods and how we arrived at our Menu for Life program balance of foods for maximum nutrient density. Because while it is a very good thing to begin eating less of the foods that you eat so that you can bring your calories in line with the Menu for Life 1,800, 2,100, or 2,400 daily calorie targets, and while is it essential to understand how to identify and work with your emotional eating issues, you also need to begin eating foods that are *better for you*.

Okay, we hear you! *Better for you?* When you hear this phrase it usually signals something distinctly unappealing, like taking medicine. But hear this: *Eating better is the most appealing and enjoyable part of the Menu for Life nutritional program!* Do you have to make changes? Yes. Do you have to give up your favorites? No! Think of it this way, you are expanding your food awareness so that you can eat what you like, add new foods as well, and eat it all in the correct proportions and with the optimal nutritional composition that promotes and supports healthful balance.

If you already started walking your 30 for 5 (see Chapter 7) and are experiencing the physical benefits of increased energy and vitality that come with moving, then it should be easy to understand that by giving your body the highest quality Energy In, you'll have the best fuel to spend as Energy Out. Not walking yet? Why wait? You know the saying, *today is the first day of the rest of your life*. We're rolling our eyes too, but *life* is what we are talking about here. A *long* life. *Your* long life. Watching your children grow up, graduate from school, settle down and start a good home. Having the opportunity to do the things you always wanted to do. Moving and eating are the essence of survival, of living. Let's take a look at what you need to do to get the highest quality for your Energy In.

DONNA RANDALL

"As soon as someone tells you that you can't have something—that becomes exactly what you want and *must* have. When it comes to food, this is particularly true if you are on that emotional roller coaster, that cycle of obesity where emotions trigger eating and eating triggers emotions. Because you want to please yourself—you haven't been able to please yourself in any other way than with the food you eat. So when everyone says to you 'This is not right, that is not right,' and the stress is building up, you eat. You eat without regard to what you are eating, when you are eating, where you are eating, how much you are eating. All that matters to you in this situation is *that* you are eating.

"Do you want to know what happens when you begin to follow your Menu for Life? You start to really get into *planning* the food you are eating, you care about eating healthfully, eating the right foods in the right proportions, and you understand that eating properly helps *reduce* your stress, even as you are losing inches and pounds and walking your '30 for 5.' Instead of a false comfort, planning, shopping, cooking, and eating the Menu for Life way becomes a *true* comfort.

"Worried about cooking? Cooking is *easy*. Cooking is *fun*. You'll create wonderful meals in no time and with little effort once you get used to doing it. *Really*. Want to make your friends and family *think* you were in the kitchen all day? That's easy too. Get yourself a cup of flour, a cup of water, and just before you serve your meal, you take some flour and throw it on your shirt, take some water and throw it on your forehead, and you come out and, you know . . . the food artist presents a Menu for Life masterpiece! Now, instead of worrying about your eating, everyone will be asking you to share your recipes. They'll be commenting on that sparkle in your eyes and how wonderful you look. You'll know you feel beautiful inside and out and every-one else will see it too. So plan, cook, eat, and share your Menu for Life—there's enough here for everyone to go home full, satisfied, healthy, and happy."

DR. RANDALL

"Everyone can lose weight. It is not impossible. But there are some barriers that keep people from doing it. Most people know, though they may not want to admit it, that they are eating too much and not getting enough activity and exercise. People will come to me and say, 'Dr. Randall, I know I need to eat certain foods or avoid certain foods because of my high blood pressure or my diabetes or because I need to lower my cholesterol, but the diets are confusing or I don't like what they are telling me to eat. What can I do?'

"The guidelines some nutritionists give patients to lose weight can be confusing. You need a couple of computers to follow them. People have trouble with the food pyramid too and I don't blame them. It's a pretty pic-ture with a lot of things on it, but what does it mean and how do you use it when you are deciding what to eat for dinner? If you eat according to the Menu for Life program, you can throw all the lists away. Everyone in your family can eat the same meals and meet their health and nutritional require-ments, while losing pounds at a safe pace and keeping the weight off."

You are eating a lot of food right now, too much food—most likely one-and-one-half to two times as much food as your body requires to fuel its Energy In needs. You know you eat too much, but you also know that how much you eat is what it takes to make you feel full. But *is it?* Or is it that you eat as much as you do right now because that is the amount of food you are used to eating. With Menu for Life, we show you how to *rebalance your plate* so you are eating less total food, while eating more of the foods that are good for you, foods that fill you up faster and make you feel bet-ter all the way around.

The first thing people say when they start eating the Menu for Life way is: *"That's not enough food for me!"* They have trouble believing there is enough food on the plate to satisfy. But after only a short time of eating balanced, nutrient-dense meals people realize, to their amazement, that the food we are giving them is almost *too much food.* It is a wonderful moment when we see that "ah-hah" look on people's faces, when they understand that they can eat good foods in the correct portion sizes and those foods will fill them up, keep them full, and fuel their activities for their best health and well-being. Why eat only one slice of stuffed crust sausage pizza when you can have a whole turkey sandwich, fresh salad, plus a delicious dessert for your lunch meal and still stay on track for your daily calorie targets?

For our Obesity Study, we had participants start the program by staying a full week at our research center unit in the hospital. They ate the nutritious, well-balanced portion-appropriate meals that we prepared for them. They went to classes to learn about nutrition and exercise, and they talked with each other and our staff in small groups to explore and understand some of the reasons they weighed so much. "I looked at what was on my plate that first night and I thought, *I am never going to make it on this little bit of food!*" says Cedric Williams. "The food seemed like a smaller amount than you can have on some fad diets. But after just a couple days, it was more food than I could eat. My problem was—before I started Menu for Life I just didn't know when to stop eating or even what I really *should* be eating to feel full in a healthy way. I wasn't hungry, and the taste wasn't it. I just didn't know about *enough*. In the study, I learned how much I was supposed to eat, how smaller quantities of better foods fill me up faster and make me feel better, and how to make all this fit my lifestyle."

FILL UP ON FOODS THAT ARE NUTRIENT DENSE

So far in talking about your Menu for Life we've discussed the energy nutrients in food—carbohydrate, protein, and fat—and how these energy nutrients contain caloric values that fuel your Energy Out. We've learned that combining these energy nutrients in the proper proportions maximizes health. So, right away, we need to look at what kinds of foods fit each energy nutrient category and work to rebalance what is on our plates to match these proportions. Doing this is trickier than it might seem at first glance because the nutritional values of convenience and processed foods may be different than what you'd expect by looking at the package advertising. (Another reason why is it better to avoid these foods when possible!) Later in this chapter, we show you how to read and compare the food labels on processed foods, which is the *only* true way to figure out their accurate nutritional content.

Foods contain more than just energy nutrients with caloric values; they also contain non-energy nutrients: vitamins and minerals. The non-energy nutrients foods provide give your body the substances necessary to repair, maintain, and build the many structures that keep your body functioning, such as blood cells and bone tissue. Vitamins, minerals, and water are essential for life. The Recommended Dietary Allowance (RDA), tells you how much of each non-energy nutrient your body requires each day to meet its health needs. Many food products, especially breads and other products made from grains, such as cereals and pasta, are fortified with vitamins and minerals to make sure you get adequate amounts of them. Fruits and vegetables have the highest non-energy nutrient content when they are eaten raw.

When foods have a high ratio of nutrient value to energy value, that is, when they deliver more non-energy nutrients at lower caloric values, the foods are *nutrient dense*. Your body loves nutrient-dense foods. These are the foods that make eating worthwhile. They deliver the nutrients that give your body its get-up-and-go. You feel more energized after eating nutrient-dense meals because you *are*—the energy mix is right for your body's Energy In/Energy Out needs.

Foods that provide little nutrient density are high in caloric values and low in non-energy nutrients. When you eat these foods, you eat meals that fail to meet the right proportions of energy nutrients or the right quantity of them. You eat lots of calories but your body is undernourished, so you eat more and more food as your body asks you to give it the nutrition it craves. But all the food delivers are "empty" calories—calories with low nutrient density.

How you prepare foods affects their nutrient density. Pasta by itself is mostly carbohydrate, an energy nutrient. Although pasta is fortified to contain some vitamins and minerals, the ratio of non-energy nutrients to energy nutrients is low—in other words, pasta by itself delivers more calories than nutrients and is a low nutrient density food.

So by itself, pasta has low nutrient density. When you add fresh or frozen vegetables and a tomato-based sauce to pasta, you create a dish that now includes the vitamins, minerals, and other non-energy nutrients that these high nutrient density foods provide. The overall nutrient density of the meal increases—you get a lot of non-energy nutrients for the calories you consume.

However, when you prepare a packaged pasta kit that comes with a sauce mix and added flavors, you end up with a dish that remains low in nutrient density because these substances add mostly fat and other non-energy nutrients but little in the way of vitamins and minerals. The overall nutrient density of this packaged pasta meal actually *decreases*—you get very little non-energy nutrients and far more calories than if you ate plain pasta.

When you eat meals that you prepare yourself with fresh ingredients, you get high nutrient value for a lower calorie cost. When you eat meals made from processed ingredients and kits—boxed, frozen, ready-to-eat, or ready-to-prepare—you get little nutrient value and lots of calories. *Most packaged food products have low nutrient density* (and are high in sodium, a potential health problem we'll talk more about later in this chapter).

Eating nutrient-dense foods in the proper portion sizes and energy nutrient proportions leaves you feeling full. These foods taste good and are good for you. As your body adjusts to the higher quality of this nutrient-dense Energy In, the way you feel inside and out improves. When you eat the *right* foods your body prompts you to eat *less food* over all, and you find yourself empowered physically and mentally through the good foods you are eating. You may find you are still challenged by emotional eating issues, but you will also find you are stronger to deal with them and less at the mercy of your food choices. Increasingly, *you* are in control of your eating. The whole concept of *enough* food becomes manageable. You know when enough food is enough. And you no longer want *or need* more.

Let's compare foods of high, moderate, and low nutrient densities in the chart on pages 156 and 157.

"When I went to the grocery store after the first week in the Obesity Study, I didn't know what to buy," says Marie Primas-Bradshaw. "All the things I always put in my basket, the high-fat foods, the salty snacks, the real butter, I couldn't do that anymore. I could see that I had to change the way I shop for food altogether. The Menu for Life program helped teach me how to transform my ways of cooking and eating. I used to have a sandwich with lots of mayonnaise and rare roast beef and cheese; then I learned to have maybe a half sandwich with some vegetables, a salad, lots of water—and I realized that made me full.

"I started measuring everything," Marie says, "so I learned how much my familiar glasses and bowls really hold. I discovered I sometimes ate at least twice as much and mistakenly thought that amount equaled one serving! When I went to restaurants, the portions were so big, too big.

Gradually I found other foods I like just as much. A lot of it is making up your mind that new foods and flavors can be good too—you can't be so picky. Or, *really*, you *can* be as picky, but now you can be picky about foods that are *good* for you."

Food Group	High Nutrient Density (Best Choices)	Moderate Nutrient Density (Acceptable Choices)	Low Nutrient Density (Empty Calories)
Grains and grain products (bread, cereal, rice, pasta)	Whole grains such as brown rice, oatmeal, shredded wheat, couscous, polenta Fortified whole grain breads including tortillas, bagels, pita bread Pastas including spaghetti noodles and macaroni	White rice Biscuits, muffins, cornbread, breadsticks Pancakes, waffles, french toast (made from scratch or mix) Granola Sweetened breakfast cereals	Cookies, cakes, pies, doughnuts, croissants Premade garlic bread Frozen waffles and pancakes Packaged macaroni and cheese products Fried rice
Vegetables	Fresh or frozen: Broccoli, cauliflower, cabbage, kale, bok choy, brussels sprouts, kohlrabi Carrots, radishes, turnips, parsnips, onions, scallions Cucumbers, squash, eggplant Greens (mustard, collard, turnip, not fried) Corn, green beans, peas, snow peas, asparagus Okra Seaweed Salad greens (butter, red, romaine lettuces), endive, escarole, baby spinach Mushrooms	Vegetables sautéed in olive oil Candied yams (sweet potatoes) Vegetables with reduced fat dips Salads with reduced fat dressings Iceberg lettuce Canned vegetables of any kind	Vegetables that are fried, including fried tomatoes, fried greens, french fries, tempura vegetables, breaded and fried mushrooms Vegetables in cheese sauces (au gratin or scalloped) or butter sauces Vegetables served with high fat dips Salads with high fat dressings and condiments Canned creamed corn
Fruits	Apples, apricots, bananas, peaches, pears, plums	Canned fruit in syrup Frozen fruits that are sweetened	Dried fruit, including raisins, prunes, and coconut

Food Group	High Nutrient Density (Best Choices)	Moderate Nutrient Density (Acceptable Choices)	Low Nutrient Density (Empty Calories)
Fruits continued	Melons, watermelon, cantaloupe Grapefruit, lemons, limes Berries Grapes Papaya, mangoes, guava Unsweetened fruit juice	Sweetened fruit juices that are at least 50% fruit juice	Olives "Fruit" juices that are less than 50% juice, fruit-flavored drinks that have no fruit juice Fruit rolls, fruit chews
Dairy (milk, yogurt, cheese)	Nonfat or 1% milk, yogurt, cheese, cottage cheese, buttermilk, sour cream Soy milk	2% milk, yogurt, cheese, cottage cheese, buttermilk, sour cream Ice milk, sherbet, sorbet	Whole milk, yogurt, cheese, cottage cheese, buttermilk, sour cream Ice cream, milkshakes Custards
Meat, poultry, fish, dry beans, eggs, and nuts	Skinless white meat chicken, turkey, game hen Fish, shellfish (not fried) Soybeans and soy products Lentils Red, navy, pinto, kidney, garbanzo beans Nonfat refried beans Tuna canned in water Lean cuts of beef and pork (USDA Select or Choice, all visible fat trimmed) Extra lean (less than 10% fat) ground beef Veal, lamb	Eggs Tuna canned in oil Ground turkey or chicken Tofu, tempeh Prime grades of beef trimmed of visible fat, prime rib Lean ground beef (less than 15% fat), corned beef Canadian bacon	Breaded and fried fish and shellfish Processed lunch meats (such as bologna, salami, pastrami) Traditional refried beans Hotdogs (all kinds) Meatloaf Regular ground beef Bacon, saltback, side pork Spareribs Sausage, bratwurst, knockwurst
Fats, oils, and sweets	None	Fatfree cooking spray Olive oil (in small amounts) Ketchup, mustard, reduced fat mayonnaise, reduced fat salad dressings	Margarine, cooking oils, lard, salad dressings, mayonnaise, avocados, Candy Soda

EATING FOR NUTRITIONAL BALANCE:
ENERGY AND NON-ENERGY NUTRIENTS

So the foods you eat have both energy value and nutritional value for your body. Let's take a closer look at each category of energy and non-energy nutrient and how and why those nutrients are important to your health and well-being.

Dietary carbohydrate. This exists in foods in the forms of sugars, starches, and fiber. Dietary carbohydrate is abundant in fruits, vegetables, and grains. Carbohydrate also "hides out" in processed foods. Manufacturers use starches and sugars to add texture, flavor, consistency, and thickness to food products—to cover for the fact that these products don't have any of these qualities on their own. This is "help" you can do without. The added carbohydrates in processed convenience foods are empty calories, because most packaged foods have low nutrient density. Raw broccoli, however, is low calorie, nutrient-dense, high-fiber carbohydrate—the kind you want to have.

Carbohydrates that enter your body as simple sugars pass through your metabolism in a fast and straight path. Glucose, being the simplest such structure, goes from food to fuel within minutes. Other basic sugar forms combine two or more glucose molecules to create structures such as sucrose, fructose, maltose, and lactose.

Other carbohydrate structures are more complex, containing multiple molecules arranged in different forms. These are starches and fiber. Starches are storage forms of sugars contained in plant-based foods such as vegetables, fruits, and grains. When you eat these foods, your body takes the storage structures apart to create the single molecules it can use for fuel. Dietary starches take longer than dietary sugars to metabolize, but still make it into your body as fuel within two to six hours. Your body can convert all of the starches from your diet into sugars. The dietary sugars you eat give your body instant carbohydrate-based fuel; starches provide smaller amounts of carbohydrate-based fuel over a longer period of time.

Fiber is what gives plants their structure. The human body cannot break down fiber into sugars for use as fuel. Fiber provides the bulk that aids in digestion by helping to move digestive waste through your intestines. High-fiber foods take longer to digest, helping you to feel full and satisfied for several hours after eating them. Fiber extends the availability of sugars over eight to twelve hours, and can help to control blood sugar and cholesterol levels when consistently included in the diet.

This three-level structure of sugar availability—the burst from basic sugars, the more sustained release of sugar from starch, and the extended release of sugar from foods high in fiber—helps your body to maintain a relatively steady level of glucose for its energy needs.

Eating the right amount of carbohydrate to maintain a steady and healthful blood glucose level is important because of the relationship between glucose and insulin. Insulin is the chemical "key" that lets glucose into, or keeps glucose out of, your cells. Eating more than 60 percent carbohydrates puts big spikes of sugar into your system. In response, your body releases big spikes of insulin to bring the sugar level back into balance again. But because the insulin response is slower than the sugar response, by the time your body sends the signal to stop releasing insulin, there is more of it in your blood than there is glucose for it to act on. Your glucose level drops to the point where it triggers hunger, making your body erroneously think you need to eat even *more* excessive carbohydrates. Over time this erratic cycle can burn out your body's normal responses, resulting in pre-diabetes or insulin resistance (your cells require greater amounts of insulin before they allow glucose to enter) and setting the stage for diabetes (type 2). Controlling your carbohydrate intake, particularly from processed foods, and eating foods high in fiber is essential to reduce your risk of developing diabetes (type 2).

Dietary protein. This exists in foods in the form of amino acids. Amino acids are important to your body because they are the basic building blocks for making and repairing cells and tissues. Your body disassembles the proteins in foods to create a "warehouse" of amino acids. It draws from this supply to reassemble amino acids into the forms it needs.

When we think of high-protein foods, we tend to think of meats because meats are the most common source of dietary protein in the American diet. The problem with this is that meats also contain dietary fat. When you meet your body's protein needs entirely from meat sources, you get too much fat. Most foods from plant sources—such as legumes, nuts, seeds, and many fruits, vegetables, and grains—contain protein too. These foods are more nutrient-dense than meats, giving your body greater value for the energy "price."

Foods that are mostly protein also satisfy your need to feel full after eating. The molecules of amino acids are very complex, so protein takes a longer time than either carbohydrate or fat for your body to digest and metabolize. A skinless, broiled chicken breast (low fat) will hold you longer than a large piece of bread or serving of pasta, both of which are primarily carbohydrate. Remember, though, that in the end protein, like fat and carbohydrate, is just another energy source to your body. When you eat more of it than your body needs, protein becomes Excess Energy—stored body fat.

You might have heard that the way to build muscle is to eat a lot of protein, especially meat. This is a myth. Your body uses amino acids to build new muscle, this much is true. But what you eat as protein, your body takes apart into amino acids. It then reassembles these amino acids to build the protein structures it needs. Dietary protein does not go directly to body protein. And it is exercise that causes your body to need more muscle—so if you *really* want to build muscle start walking your 30 for 5. No matter how much protein you eat, your body uses only what it needs and considers the remainder as excess.

Dietary fat. This exists in foods in the forms of lipids such as fatty acids, triglycerides, and cholesterol. *Fat, itself, is not bad—or bad for you.* Your body needs a certain amount of lipids to carry out many of its functions. What is bad about fat is that most of us eat too much of it, which means it becomes Excess Energy. Unlike carbohydrate and protein, which require your body to spend energy to turn them into energy forms and fuel, dietary fat is very easy for your body to metabolize because it does not break down into further components after digestion. Whatever fatty acids remain in your bloodstream without being called on for fuel go straight to fat cells for storage. They get called back only when your Activity Energy Out needs exceed the amount of available energy sources in your body.

In nature, dietary fat almost always exists in combination with protein, such as in meats and dairy products. Foods from plant sources that contain fat, such as soybeans, are also high in protein. This is nature's way of balancing how much fat you eat. In these combinations, the proportions of fat and protein are remarkably close to the proportions that are ideal for health. Unfortunately, most of the fat you eat does not come from nature, but from fried and processed foods. These are foods that have low nutrient density—nearly all processed, fast food, and carryout foods. And beware labels that proclaim the product contains less fat in some way because this is only in relation to the "full" fat version. Such foods still contain fat, and you must read the label carefully to determine how much. Look also at the carbohydrates. Many products with less fat also contain more sugar, which your body will convert to fat when the sugar is unused as Energy Out.

Label Claim	What It Means	Comments
Fat-free, no fat, nonfat, zero fat	Contains less than 1/2 (0.5) gram of fat per serving	Consuming more than one serving size can easily give you a hefty portion of fat
Lowfat, low in fat	Contains less than 3 grams of fat per serving	Consuming more than one serving significantly boosts fat content
Less fat, reduced fat	Contains 25 percent or less fat per serving compared to the "full fat" version of the product	Read the label to determine the actual fat content per serving; comparing to the "full fat" product gives you no useful information
Light	Contains 50 percent or less fat per serving compared to the "full fat" version of the product	Read the label to determine the actual fat content per serving; comparing to the "full fat" product gives you no useful information
Lean	Meats and poultry that contain less than 10 grams of fat per 3-ounce serving	Consuming more than one serving size significantly boosts fat content
Extra lean	Meats and poultry that contain less than 5 grams of fat per 3-ounce serving	Consuming more than one serving size significantly boosts fat content

Water and Alcohol. Alcohol is another energy nutrient. Water is a non-energy nutrient. Water is essential to life; alcohol is not. Alcohol contains an energy value of seven calories per ounce—seven *empty* calories per ounce. When planning meals to meet your daily Menu for Life calorie targets of 1,800, 2,100, and 2,400, you need to consider the number of calories in that glass of wine with dinner or that beer you drink in front of the television late at night. Consider empty calories from alcohol as carefully as you consider the empty calories in a fast food meal. Are they *really* worth it?

Water has zero calories and is the most important nourishing substance you put into your body. Without water, you die. Water hydrates your body and makes it possible for all of life's functions to take place. You need about 12 cups—72 ounces—of water every day. About half of this water comes from the foods you eat. This means you should drink at least six cups of water during the day. Do you think you do? *Drink as much water as you want.* Water helps you feel full, refreshed, and invigorated.

Vitamins. These are organic nutrients. They come from living sources (except when you buy them in a bottle from the store). Vitamins create chemical actions that make it possible for your cells to use the energy available to them in your body and also have numerous health benefits. There are 13 common vitamins your body needs. Nine of them are water-soluble—they dissolve in water. Your body draws what it needs from water-soluble vitamins and then passes the excess from your body. You need to get enough of these vitamins every day. The other four are fat-soluble—they only dissolve in fatty acids. Your body stores fat-soluble vitamins in fat tissue and draws from its supplies when it needs the vitamins. You need to have an adequate amount of fat-soluble vitamins in your body, but you don't need to consume them every day. Because your body continues to store fat-soluble vitamins even when it has enough, it is possible to accumulate too much, and this *over*storage sometimes causes health problems.

Overcooking, cooking in the microwave, and exposure to air all can cause water-soluble vitamins to lose much of their nutritional value. Broil

VITAMIN	HOW YOUR BODY USES	FOOD SOURCES
Water-Soluble		
Thiamin (Vitamin B1)	Energy metabolism; aids functions of nerve and muscle cells	Fortified cereals and breads, rice, pasta, peas, corn, potatoes, oranges, watermelon, milk, beans (kidney, pinto, garbanzo), pork, ham
Riboflavin (Vitamin B2)	Energy metabolism	Fortified cereals and breads, broccoli, spinach, peas, bananas, milk, yogurt, cottage cheese, mushrooms, clams, beef, chicken, fish
Niacin (Vitamin B3)	Energy metabolism, especially glucose and fat	Fortified cereals and breads, spinach, potatoes, milk, cottage cheese, peanut butter, beans (kidney, pinto, garbanzo), sunflower seeds, chicken, beef, fish, canned tuna, shrimp, tofu

VITAMIN	HOW YOUR BODY USES	FOOD SOURCES
Pyridoxine (Vitamin B6)	Amino acid metabolism	Fortified breads and cereals, broccoli, carrots, potatoes, sweet potatoes, bananas, watermelon, avocados, sunflower seeds, beef, chicken, turkey, fish, tuna
Cyanacobalamine (Vitamin B12)	Energy metabolism; aids in functions of nerve and muscle cells; essential for new cells	Animal-based foods: meats, poultry, eggs, milk, cheese; fortified soy milk
Biotin	Energy metabolism, especially fatty acids and amino acids	Fortified breads and cereals, eggs, many vegetables and fruits
Pantothenic Acid	Energy metabolism; hormone production; aids in functions of nerve and muscle cells	Fortified breads and cereals, potatoes, tomatoes, broccoli, beef, chicken
Folate (Folic Acid)	Energy metabolism; helps prevent neural tube defects in early pregnancy	Fortified breads and cereals, spinach, broccoli, peas, corn, oranges, avocados, beans (kidney, pinto, garbanzo), tofu, lentils, asparagus, turnip greens
Vitamin C	Antioxidant that helps protect against illness and disease; aids in healing	Broccoli, sweet potatoes, potatoes, tomato juice, oranges, strawberries, watermelon, grapefruit and grapefruit juice, red bell peppers, mangoes, brussels sprouts
Fat-Soluble		
Vitamin A	Health of the eyes, connective tissues, skin; general growth	Fortified breads and cereals, carrots, spinach, sweet potatoes, milk, cheese, shrimp, eggs, mangoes, turnip greens
Vitamin D	Health of the bones and teeth	Sunlight; fortified milk
Vitamin E	Antioxidant that helps protect against illness and disease; aids in healing	Spinach, turnip greens, eggs, nuts, sunflower and other seeds
Vitamin K	Blood clotting; aids in building new bone	Spinach, broccoli, cauliflower, cabbage, kale, fortified milk

meats and poultry and steam your vegetables to preserve the highest level of nutrients in these foods. Better yet, eat your vegetables raw. Canned and processed vegetables lose much of their nutritional value through the canning process, which requires high temperatures to kill bacteria.

Minerals. These are inorganic nutrients. They come from nonliving sources. Minerals aid in many body functions, and your body needs different minerals in varying amounts. Minerals stay in foods through most cooking processes. The exception is when you boil foods, such as vegetables, in water—the water draws the minerals out, so when you throw the water down the drain most of the minerals go with it. Steam vegetables— the moist heat cooks the vegetables to the right tenderness, yet preserves the minerals so your body gets them.

Some minerals, such as chloride, potassium, and sodium, are in the form of salts and usually in combinations such as sodium chloride. This refers more to their chemical structures than to the taste sensations they activate. The only time a salt form tastes salty is when it contains chloride; table salt is a combination of sodium (40 percent) and chloride (60 percent). A few drops of lemon juice can take the place of salt when what you are after is the salt taste.

MINERALS	HOW YOUR BODY USES	FOOD SOURCES
Calcium	Build and maintain bones and teeth; regulates muscle contractions including of the heart	Milk, cheese, yogurt, spinach, kale, bok choy, turnip greens, broccoli, tofu, canned sardines with bones, anchovies with bones, shrimp, almonds, oranges, fortified orange juice, kidney, navy, pinto, garbanzo beans
Chloride	Regulates fluid balances in the body; forms digestive acids	Salt, soy sauce, processed foods, meat, milk, eggs
Chromium	Aids in insulin/glucose interactions	Beef, pork, ham, chicken, turkey, eggs, cheese, whole grains and whole grain products
Copper	Aids in energy metabolism and immune functions	Salmon, mushrooms, nuts, oatmeal, whole grains and whole grain products, kidney, navy, pinto, garbanzo beans, sunflower seeds, peanuts
Iodine	Essential to produce thyroid hormones that regulate metabolism	Iodized salt, all fish and shellfish, almonds, processed foods to which iodine is added

MINERALS	HOW YOUR BODY USES	FOOD SOURCES
Iron	Transport of oxygen from lungs to cells throughout the body	Fortified breads and cereals, spinach, peas, carrots, green beans, parsley, tomatoes, potatoes, kidney, navy, pinto, garbanzo beans; shrimp, fish, beef, ham, pork, clams, raisons, watermelon
Magnesium	Energy metabolism; build and maintain bones and teeth; new cell and tissue growth; assists muscle and nerve cell functions	"Hard" water, spinach, broccoli, potatoes, parsnips, lima beans, milk, yogurt, kidney, navy, pinto, garbanzo beans; fish, nuts, seeds, beef, ham, pork, chicken, turkey, artichoke, fortified breads and cereals
Manganese	Assists in many metabolic functions	Nuts, spinach, okra, kale, pineapple, strawberries, tea, whole grains and whole grain products, lentils
Phosphorus	Energy metabolism; new cell and tissue growth; build and maintain bones and teeth	Milk, yogurt, cheese, cottage cheese, kidney, navy, pinto, garbanzo beans; tofu, beef, fish, chicken, turkey, nuts, seeds, processed foods especially lunchmeats
Potassium	Regulates fluid balances in the body; essential for muscle and nerve cell functions	Processed foods, all vegetables especially squash, potatoes, sweet potatoes, carrots, broccoli, spinach, tomatoes, okra, squash, artichokes; all fruits, especially bananas, strawberries, oranges, watermelon, grapefruit, avocado; kidney, navy, pinto, garbanzo beans; fish especially cod; beef, ham, chicken, turkey, tofu, seeds and nuts, peanut butter, milk, yogurt
Selenium	Aids in thyroid hormone production	Chicken, turkey, brown rice, eggs, peanuts, fish, shellfish
Sodium	Regulates fluid balances in the body; essential for muscle and nerve cell functions	Salt, soy sauce, processed foods, packaged cereals, bread, baked goods, beef, ham, pork, milk, all vegetables
Sulfur	Necessary for the functions of proteins and vitamins	Beef, chicken, turkey, ham, pork, fish, eggs, nuts, kidney, navy, pinto, garbanzo beans
Zinc	Essential for healing, sperm development, insulin manufacture, and growth and development	Fortified breads and cereals, wheat bran, wheat germ, peas, milk, yogurt, cheese, peanut butter, kidney, navy, pinto, garbanzo beans; beef, shrimp, tofu, ham, pork, tuna, chicken, turkey, oysters, crab, avocado

You don't need very much sodium to meet your body's needs—some studies say as little as 115 milligrams a day, although the accepted *minimum* in the United States that we follow is 500 milligrams a day. Like dietary fat, dietary sodium is not by itself bad or bad for you. It becomes a problem only when your diet contains too much of it—a point that is easy to reach in today's environment of processed foods. Salt has been the world's favorite preservative since the beginning of civilization, and even with all of our modern food processing methods, this remains true. Nearly every processed and packaged food contains sodium as a preservative.

Because so many foods now contain high amounts of sodium, we have learned much about the health problems associated with eating too much of it. The most significant is high blood pressure. Sodium—salt—attracts fluid. In your body, what this means is that your blood carries more water than usual, so your heart has to work harder to push this extra volume through your arteries. In some people, this extra pressure stays high. So in our Menu for Life, we have an upper limit for sodium: 2,000 milligrams. This level is more than adequate for your body's needs, yet not so high, for most people, to cause health problems.

When we talk about cutting back on the salt that you eat, do you think about the white stuff you sprinkle on your food? One teaspoonful of table salt equals 2,000 milligrams of sodium! Salt you add to your food during cooking or at the table accounts for approximately 15 percent of the sodium most people consume. Processed foods, because they are preserved, account for the largest amount of sodium—60 to 75 percent—you put into your body. Canned foods, processed lunchmeats, snack chips and crackers, dill pickles, and instant puddings contain very high amounts of sodium. So does soda. You need to read food labels carefully to watch for excessive amounts of sodium in the products you buy. Entrees with more than 800 mg of sodium should be avoided. A low-sodium food has 140 mg or less per serving.

"I used to love salt," says Clarence White. "Now I don't know when I last used salt. I read the food labels, stay away from saturated fats and foods with high sodium content. I stay away too from prepared foods. I eat mostly chicken, turkey, a little fish, vegetables. I really can't seem to get into fruits, but vegetables, yes! I drink a lot more water than I used to. I live alone and cook for myself. Exercise—I'm retired Army and I've always known exercise is important. So that part of Menu for Life made sense to me right away. Learning about the amounts and types of foods to eat, I needed to know more about. But once you learn it, you live it!"

A Little Help from the Labels

As much as possible, buy and eat fresh foods, especially vegetables and fruits. Most other foods in our country come in packages, and federal law requires that packaged foods contain food labels that provide specific and consistent information about the food's nutritional content. Most packaged foods must contain a "Nutrition Facts" panel on the label that tells you:

- The serving size and the number of servings in the package or container.
- How many calories worth of energy each serving provides, and what percentage of these calories comes from fat. This helps you to identify hidden fats.
- The amounts of key nutrients each serving provides, reported in "% Daily Values" or "% DV." This gives you a way to assess what it means when a food has a particular nutrient content and how this content counts toward meeting your daily needs for the nutrient.
- The energy value (measured in calories) and the energy sources each serving provides.
- The amount of sodium each serving provides.
- Specific nutrients: vitamin A, vitamin C, calcium, and iron. Manufacturers can choose to list other nutrients.
- Ingredients—everything that is in the product, listed in order of greatest to least quantity by weight. The closer to the head of the list you find substances such as sugars and syrups, the more of these substances the product contains (and the lower its nutrient density).

Nutrition Facts

| Serving Size | About 24 biscuits (59g/2.1oz.) |
| Servings per Container | About 28 |

| | | Cereal with 1/2 Cup Vitamins A&D |
Amount Per Serving	Cereal	Fat Free Milk
Calories	200	240
Calories from Fat	10	10

	% Daily Value**	
Total Fat 1g*	2%	2%
Saturated Fat 0g	0%	0%
Monounsaturated Fat 0g		
Polyunsaturated Fat 0.5g		
Cholesterol 0mg	0%	0%
Sodium 5mg	0%	3%
Potassium 200mg	6%	12%
Total Carbohydrate 48g	16%	18%
Dietary Fiber 6g	24%	24%
Sugars 12g		
Other Carbohydrate 30g		
Protein 6g		

Vitamin A	0%	4%
Vitamin C	0%	2%
Calcium	0%	15%
Iron	90%	90%
Thiamin	25%	30%
Riboflavin	25%	35%
Niacin	25%	25%
Vitamin B6	25%	25%
Folic Acid	25%	25%
Vitamin B12	25%	35%
Phosphorus	15%	25%
Magnesium	15%	20%
Zinc	10%	15%
Copper	10%	10%

* Amount in cereal. One half cup of fat free milk contributes an additional 40 calories, 65mg sodium, 6g total carbohydrate (6g sugars), and 4g protein.
** Percent Daily Values are based on a 2,000 calorie diet. Your daily values may be higher or lower depending on your calorie needs:

	Calories	2,000	2,500
Total Fat	Less than	65g	80g
Sat. Fat	Less than	20g	25g
Cholesterol	Less than	300mg	300mg
Sodium	Less than	2,400mg	2,400mg
Potassium		3,500mg	3,500mg
Total Carbohydrate		300g	375g
Dietary Fiber		25g	30g

Calories per gram: Fat 9 • Carbohydrate 4 • Protein 4

Ingredients: Whole grain wheat, sugar, sorbitol, gelatin, **Vitamins and Minerals:** reduced iron, niacinamide, zinc oxide, pyridoxine hydrochloride (vitamin B6), riboflavin (vitamin B2), thiamin hydrochloride (vitamin B1), folic acid and vitamin B12. To maintain quality, BHT has been added to the packaging.

CONTAINS WHEAT INGREDIENTS.

Exchange: 2 ½ Carbohydrates
The dietary exchanges are based on the *Exchange Lists for Meal Planning*, ©1995 by The American Diabetes Association, Inc. and The American Dietetic Association.

Food Label

Food labels also include a chart showing the Daily Values typical for food intake at the 2000-calorie and 2500-calorie levels and tell you the number of calories per gram for the three energy sources. For your Menu for Life, we recommend an 1800-calorie, 2100-calorie, or 2400-calorie level, according to your needs, so you can better manage your Energy In.

Despite this regimented structure, manufacturers manage to find enough leeway to make their products look as good as possible nutritionally. Examine these labels for breakfast cereal. Which cereal appears to offer the greatest nutrient density?

The cereal on the left, Cereal A, has fewer calories, and no calories from fat. Does that make it the more nutritious choice? Not necessarily! First, it's a smaller serving size. Will you feel full when you eat this amount or will you be tempted to have twice or three times as much? Next, look at the energy nutrients these cereals provide. The cereal on the right, Cereal B, has more than twice as much carbohydrate, including a significant percentage of fiber—18 percent of the Daily Value—to make you feel full and satisfied when you are finished eating your serving. Although both cereals have about the same amount of sugars, the Energy In from Cereal B is going to hold you well through the morning because it takes longer for your body to digest and metabolize high fiber foods. The Energy In from Cereal A comes almost entirely from sugar, which will be gone in a few hours. Now, look at the non-energy nutrients. Cereal A is going to take 10 percent of your daily sodium allocation, while Cereal B contains no sodium. Cereal B contains substantial amounts of almost twice as many non-energy nutrients as Cereal A. More important, Cereal B gives you 90 *percent* of your Daily Value for iron, an important trace element, while Cereal A gives you just 10 percent. Cereal B also gives you more than twice as much folic acid, a particularly important nutrient if there is any possibility you could become pregnant (folic acid, or folate, helps prevent neural tube defects, a group of potentially fatal birth defects). Which cereal would *you* choose for your Menu for Life?

Compare different brands of the "same" products and you'll be surprised at how different they can be. Watch for hidden additions. Read the whole label and make sure it reflects the way you actually eat the product. For example, most people add milk to cereal. Now, cereal labels offer nutrition facts to take this into account—for nonfat (or the label might say skim) milk. If you are using 1 percent or 2 percent milk, the nutritional values

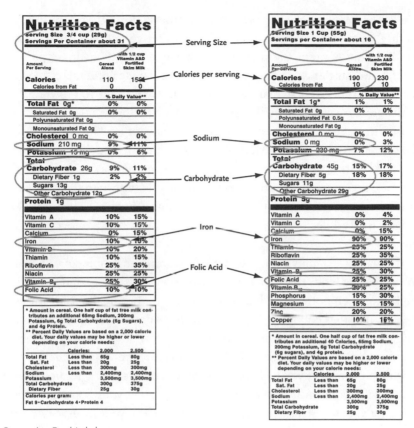

Comparing Food Labels

will be different. Packaged foods with ingredients such as pasta and a sauce mix to which you add other ingredients like margarine and milk might list the nutritional values for the *dry* product. But you don't *eat* these products dry! Make sure you understand what nutritional value you are receiving when you put convenience processed and packaged foods on your plate . . . and into your mouth.

Menu for Life Meal Planning, Shopping, and Cooking

Why let someone else decide what is in the foods you eat and how they are prepared? The only way to adopt good eating habits is to plan your meals, shop wisely, and cook for yourself and your family. In Chapter 9, you'll learn exactly how to plan a week's meals using the Menu for Life method of food exchanges. Food exchanges let you choose among foods you like that contain the proper daily balance of carbohydrate, protein, and fat, are nutrient dense, and add up to the daily calorie targets you are aiming for. Once you've planned your meals, we'll teach you how to shop in the grocery store and we'll share Donna's marvelous Menu for Life food artistry in more than 30 recipes. "It took a while for my family to adjust to the changes in food," says Alquietta Brown. "I started cooking and eating a lot of fresh vegetables instead of canned, getting away from all the starches, eating smaller portions. Now I don't add salt when I'm cooking— I use celery seed, garlic, pepper, things like that. When they all saw me lose weight, they all decided they wanted to lose weight too. So now we all eat this way."

If you are the family's cook, sometimes it works to simply start choosing and preparing foods that fit with your Menu for Life. Your family members might not even notice the change, or if they do, they might enjoy the new flavors and foods enough to give them a try. What if they resist? You can't change anyone else. You can do the best you can do to show other family members how much the changes you are making are improving your life, how much healthier you feel and look, how you are starting to drop inches and even pounds. You can show them all the good your Menu for Life is doing for you, but *you can only change yourself.* Keep your focus! Stick with the changes you know are making your life better.

What if you are not the family cook, and the person who does the shopping and the cooking doesn't want to accommodate your changes? Offer to share the cooking duties. Or, if that is not possible, do what you can to make the meals more healthful. Remove the skin from the chicken. Avoid fried foods. Request more fresh fruits and vegetables. Go grocery shopping with the cook and start reading the food labels on the products he or she wants to buy to be sure they are the wisest food choices. Be tenacious and over time you may find your input makes a difference and the cook is more interested and eager to work with you to create more healthful family meals. Ask for some of the recipes in this book!

Parties, holidays (when there is so much food and lots of high-fat desserts), eating out at restaurants or at a friend's house—these situations can be challenging for you. Don't let the challenge of them stop you from being with the family and friends you love, but don't let them interfere with your Menu for Life either. Look for the healthiest choices, and go with them. If someone says you are not eating enough, tell them you are there to celebrate, not to eat! "We eat for birthdays and anniversaries and Christmas and Thanksgiving and Easter and New Year's Day," says Stephanie Dove. "Every holiday in this country is centered around serving meals. But the focus of your life should be about more than preparing and eating food, it should be about being together and celebrating as a family."

There will be times when someone else is cooking and everything on the table is everything that you used to eat, and you just can't take the temptation. Or you are at a party and all the salads have mayonnaise and the chicken has deep-fried skin *and* gravy. Or maybe the *only* thing you want to eat is a half-gallon of ice cream, and you make your way through most or all of it even though you know you shouldn't. It's okay. You are human, and life is not perfect. "When you slip back to your old ways," says Howard Copeland, "just pick up and go right back. That is what I do. I start drinking my water again. I like tuna fish on black bread, rye bread. Eat more fresh fruit, drink 100 percent juice. Walk the 30 for 5. Get back on it. Get back on that Menu for Life. My nephew got married recently and someone at my table said to me 'You don't eat as much as you used to! You've lost some weight!' When people notice, you feel good about that."

There are ups and downs in a Menu for Life. This is what keeps it real. What is done is done. Today, you have a new balance to manage. Start the day with renewed determination. Did you overindulge at dinner last night? Get up and go for a morning walk. Put your body in motion. Enjoy the movement, the activity. Feel your muscles and tissues stretch and warm to the exercise. Remind yourself how wonderful you feel when you are doing what is right and good for your body, for your health, for yourself. In a Menu for Life, each day is a fresh beginning full of boundless opportunities. Live beautifully!

9

~~~~~~~

Your Menu for Life Meal Planner

All of those fad diets you have tried through the years . . . how many of them tell you that you can eat *anything* you want and still lose weight? Sounds good! Sounds very good. But when you start planning your meals according to the diet's instructions, you discover you are allowed to eat anything you want if it comes from the *list of foods*. And what these diets consider a "serving" looks like a tiny little bite! Other diet plans require that you eat—or not eat—certain kinds of foods. You can eat mostly high-fat foods or no fats at all. Mostly high-protein foods or no protein at all. Mostly high-carbohydrate foods or no carbohydrates at all.

Although it might be fun, for a short time, to splurge on "forbidden" foods, and at the same time see a few pounds come off, over the weeks you notice it is harder and harder to follow the diet's rules. You find yourself struggling to stick to the diet—if only because it is restrictive to be a fol-lower forever! The fad diet feels boring, unsatisfying. You get tired of hav-ing to eat a certain type of food all the time, or prepare foods in a bland style, or of thinking all the time: is this a "yes" food or a "no" food. How often do you just decide outright that you've lost enough weight on this diet and return, relieved, to your old, familiar way of eating? Or, without any creative input into what you are eating, you find yourself losing inter-est and falling back into old eating patterns, a little more every day until you are back where you started? Either way, the pounds creep up again.

Still other diets "conveniently" sell you prepared and packaged meals.

All you do is heat our delicious, already prepared meals in your microwave oven! Do you want some corporation to tell you what to eat for the rest of your life? Personally, we feel it is no thrill to eat out of a box. Are prepackaged meals ever as good, or as good for you, as what you can make for yourself and for your family in your own kitchen? (Try Donna's recipes if you are unsure about the answer to that question!)

It is impossible to take control of your eating if all you do is go from one fad diet to another. When every diet you try has a different approach to eating, you confuse your body . . . and your mind. And all of these kinds of diets leave you feeling deprived in some way. They take away your favorite foods, or they feed you *less* healthful variety than your body needs to nourish and sustain itself. You feel hungry, frustrated, and unfulfilled. All you can think about is what you *can't have.* When you think about what you *can't have* all the time, you want it even more. Food is always on your mind. And any time you think about food, you want to eat—which becomes pretty much all the time.

Even the medical diets your doctor may have given you often are confusing and disappointing. When you have health problems like high blood pressure, high cholesterol, or diabetes—health problems that are linked to how and what you eat as well as to how much you weigh—you get *lists.* Your doctor, or a nutritionist, gives you *lists* of the foods you can eat and, mostly, the foods that you *can't* eat. And for every condition, the lists are different. What are you supposed to *do* with these lists? You can't eat them! What do these lists mean to you when you are trying to figure out what to eat for dinner? What's on the "yes" list for one condition shows up on the "no" list for another. Which list do you follow? If you are hungry for a burger today, you are going to follow the list that lets you have one! And what do you do about these lists if you are cooking for a whole family and not just one person on a "special" diet? Odds are good that you'll end up preparing separate meals, and that's a lot of extra work!

DONNA RANDALL

"If you can buy it—if you can see the meal you want offered in a restaurant or in a picture on the front of a frozen food box, then you can cook it yourself, and *healthfully* too. *You can.* Don't tell me that you *can't.* I know that just means that you *don't want to.*

"Before I cook anything on the stove, I cook it in my head. And if it doesn't come out . . . if I can't picture myself bringing out a perfect dish, then I scrap the idea and start thinking in a new direction. If the meal I'm conceiving comes out in my head, whether I cook it or not, I know that recipe is right. So be imaginative, and *never give up*. We all love thinking about food, so revel in creating in your mind the mouth-watering healthful meals you are going to plan and prepare for yourself and your loved ones. Revel in the time you spend in the kitchen, working with the food, preparing it with love. Serve your meals with pride, and eat with whole-hearted satisfaction—no guilt, no regrets."

DR. RANDALL

"If we had the resources, we'd take on the fast food corporations. We believe it is possible to produce the food, make it convenient, good-tasting, with greater variety, and stop obesity. That day is still somewhere in the future. Today, though, it is becoming easier for the home cook to shop and read food labels to choose the most healthful and nutritious products. It takes a lot of time and effort, but meal planning is the best way we know to help a new generation of cooks take care of their health."

You are spending a lot of time and effort on ways of eating that keep your life out of the synergy of health and well-being. And you know it. We want you to take all this hope and determination that you put into fad diets and special diets and use it once and for all to break the cycle of weight gain, emotional distress, and physical illness. We want to see you apply your efforts where you can see some lasting results.

Do the work! When you use the Menu for Life Meal Planner, you have to do some *work* to create a week's worth of healthful meals for you and your family. But learning how to build nutritious nutrient-dense, low-calorie, low-sodium meals with the Menu for Life Meal Planner puts you back in control of what you eat, when, and how much. Instead of just following, instead of just eating what's put in front of you, *you* create the meals. You plan, shop, and cook like a food artist. You are the chef in your Menu for Life! After all, the chef is the one who decides what food will be offered, who chooses and prepares the meals with love. If you eat according to the Menu for Life guidelines, you can serve the food you prepare with confidence to any family member—even those who have health concerns they need to factor into their food choices.

Don't have time to cook? *Make time.* The time you spend improving what you eat will translate into health benefits that can *extend your life!*

Remember, obesity puts you at greater risk for serious health problems. You're not the one cooking the meals? *Hand this book to the person who is doing the cooking.* Sit down together to work through the Meal Planner steps. Learn how to eat healthfully, and help your whole family in the process.

When you use the Menu for Life Meal Planner, you figure out in advance when and what you are going to eat next. You *plan* your eating. If you call food your "addiction," then why not turn this negative into a positive? Planning your week's meals gives you hours of thinking about the food you will eat. Knowing that the food you choose is good for you makes you feel good about the time you put into it. *You can feel good about the time you spend thinking about food!* There's no more need to indulge in guilty plotting over food or distracting thoughts of where or when you will eat next. No more feeling out of control in the grocery store, stuffed with packaged foods that scream their advertising at you as you walk down the aisle. You plan what you are going to eat, you make your shopping list, and you buy only what you need; *you* are in control.

To start losing weight, you need to get a handle on what and how much you *do* eat, right now. As we did in Chapter 4, we need to take a close look at your Energy In—at how much you eat. Not how much you think you eat, or want other people to believe you eat, but *how much you **really** eat.* A little later in this section, we ask you to do a food journal, to write down everything you eat, how much of it you eat, and when you eat it. From this, you will know how much food you consume each day, and where those calories come from. It will tell you *how you eat* right now. Before you do your food journal, though, we need to talk more about what food is composed of and how we can choose a variety of foods that gives us everything our body *needs*, as well as what our body *likes*, all in healthful synergy.

Menu for Life Synergy: Food Types, Food Groups, Food Exchanges

Doctors and nutritionists know what kinds of foods, and how much of them, you should eat. We know this from a science perspective, in terms of how foods affect your health and the way your body functions. We know what nutrients, and how much of them, your body requires. You know, or will know after you do your food journal, what kinds of foods, and how much of them, you like to eat. Your Menu for Life combines the two—science and what you like—into a dynamic synergy that can support your health and well-being for the rest of your life. This synergy has three parts:

- Food type
- Food group
- Food exchanges

Food type. This defines which of three energy sources make up a food's basic composition: fat, protein, and carbohydrate. To get Energy In, you need at least one of these three. Whether you receive the benefits of that energy today, tomorrow, or way on down the road after the energy has been stored as fat, depends on how much energy you take in at one time and how much energy your body uses. This is how your *body* views food. For most people, a good balance is for the calories of each day's food intake to be about 25 percent fat, 12 to 15 percent protein, and 55 to 60 percent carbohydrate.

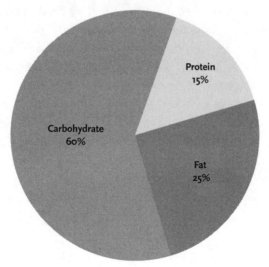

Food Type Percentages

Food group. This defines the *kinds* or categories of foods that you eat. From a science perspective, food groups organize foods according to their chemical and nutrient characteristics and structures. As you learned in Chapter 8, some foods are not really what they seem to be. (Tomatoes are in the vegetable group, but they are technically fruit.) From *your* perspective, food groups organize foods according to *how you view them*; this is what you buy and eat. There are six food groups:

- Grains and grain products (bread, cereal, rice, pasta)
- Vegetables
- Fruits
- Dairy (milk, yogurt, cheese)
- Meat, poultry, fish, dry beans, eggs, and nuts
- Fats, oils, and sweets

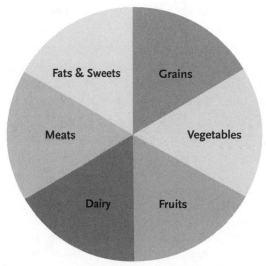

The Six Food Groups

Nearly all foods, no matter what food group they belong to, contain varying amounts of the three energy sources, fat, protein, and carbohydrate; most contain two, and many contain all three. By looking at what foods go in which food groups, you can begin to choose foods that contain more of one energy source than another.

- **Meat, poultry,** and **fish** contain mostly protein, some fat, and no carbohydrate
- **Vegetables** contain mostly carbohydrate, some protein, and no fat
  Fruits contain mostly carbohydrate and no protein or fat
- **Grain** products such as pasta and bread contain carbohydrate, protein, and fat

- **Added fats** such as butter and oil contain only fat
- **Added sweets** such as sugar, honey, and syrup contain only carbohydrate

Foods also contain other nutrients that are important for health, such as vitamins and minerals. When you select the foods you eat from among the food groups *in the recommended percentages for balanced eating*—25 percent fat, 12 to 15 percent protein, and 55 to 60 percent carbohydrate—you will get all the vitamins, minerals, and other nutrients that your body needs to maintain health and prevent disease. You will meet your RDAs (the amounts of nutrients that meet the health needs of a typical adult).

COMMON FOODS IN THE SIX FOOD GROUPS

GRAINS & GRAIN PRODUCTS	VEGETABLES	FRUITS	DAIRY	MEAT, POULTRY, FISH, DRIED BEANS, EGGS	FATS & SWEETS
Whole grains (wheat, oats, rice, barley, buckwheat, bulgur, millet, rye), flour from any grain, grits, wheat germ, cream of wheat, oatmeal, granola, cereals, breads (white, wheat, rye, sourdough, french, fancy), muffins, bagels, rolls, crackers, pasta, noodles, spaghetti,	fresh or canned asparagus, beets, green beans, wax beans, artichokes, broccoli, brussels sprouts, beets, cabbage, sauerkraut, carrots, cauliflower, celery, cucumbers, greens, kohlrabi, onions, okra, salad greens, lettuce, mushrooms, peppers, radishes,	fresh, dried, or canned apples, apricots, bananas, blueberries, cherries, strawberries, blackberries, raspberries, cantaloupe, figs, grapes, raisins, grapefruit, kiwi, melons, mangos, papayas, plums, prunes, plantains, lemons, limes, oranges, watermelon, peaches,	milk, cheese, cream, sour cream, cottage cheese, buttermilk, butter, half & half, whipped cream, eggnog, ice milk, ice cream, yogurt, custard, milkshakes, fortified soy milk	beef, pork, ham, lamb, veal, sausage, ground beef, veal, pork, ham, bacon, venison, squirrel, rabbit, duck, goose, quail, pheasant, chicken, game hen, turkey, eggs, kidney beans, pinto beans, navy beans, lima beans, black-eyed peas, chickpeas (garbanzo beans), soybeans, tofu, tempeh, soy products, nuts, hummus, tuna, salmon, catfish, trout, shrimp, scallops, clams,	shortening, vegetable oil, canola oil, corn oil, safflower oil, olive oil, peanut oil, lard, tallow, bacon grease, margarine, mayonnaise, avocados, olives, salad dressing, sugar, syrup, candy, snack cakes, pies, sweet rolls, doughnuts, jellies, jams, fruit spreads, potato and other snack chips, most gravies

COMMON FOODS IN THE SIX FOOD GROUPS

GRAINS & GRAIN PRODUCTS	VEGETABLES	FRUITS	DAIRY	MEAT, POULTRY, FISH, DRIED BEANS, EGGS	FATS & SWEETS
macaroni, linguini, rotini, pancakes, waffles, croissants, English muffins, biscuits, french toast, white rice, brown rice, instant rice, Ramen noodles	spinach, tomatoes, turnips, zucchini; tomato sauce, vegetable juices	pears; fruit juices		crab, oysters, lobster, crayfish, bluefish, halibut, haddock, cod, perch, swordfish, snapper, imitation crab (surimi), pollock, grouper, flounder	

Food exchanges. These define foods according to similarities in food value—how much energy a particular food's energy sources deliver. Food exchanges have different energy values, which we measure as calories, according to both food group and food type. This is because the food types (fat, protein, and carbohydrate) have different calorie values.

FOOD TYPE	CALORIES PER GRAM	CALORIES PER OUNCE
Carbohydrate	4	120
Protein	4	120
Fat	9	270

Planning your food exchanges lets you eat more foods with more variety selected from the different food groups. Using food exchanges gives you a way to make sure you balance the right food types by choosing foods from the food groups that you *need* as well as foods that you *like*, producing a healthful Menu for Life synergy and a balance in *total* calories. You design menus suited just for you and your family's needs, no matter what health conditions you, your loved ones, or your dinner guests, may have.

There are eight categories of food exchanges:

- **Starch**—includes breads, cereals and grains, vegetables high in starch, crackers, dried beans and peas, and starchy foods that also include fat such as baked goods
- **Other Carbohydrate**—includes foods high in concentrated sweets, such as bakery goods, candy, and desserts
- **Fruit**—includes fresh, dried, and canned fruits as well as fruit juices
- **Vegetable**—includes vegetables and products made from them such as tomato sauce and vegetable juices
- **Milk**—divided into nonfat, lowfat, reduced fat, and whole milk
- **Meat and Meat Substitutes**—includes meats, poultry, seafood, cheese, eggs, tofu; divided into very lean, lean, medium fat, and high fat
- **Fat**—includes fats, oils, and foods high in fats
- **Free Foods**—includes condiments, fat-free and reduced-fat foods, and sugar-free and reduced-sugar foods

Food Exchange Category	Food Type Energy Sources	Energy (Calorie) Value	Amounts/ Serving Sizes	Sample Foods
Starch	Carbohydrate, 15 grams Protein, 3 grams Fat, 1 gram or less	80 calories	1 ounce or 1/2 cup	bread, cornbread, muffins, rolls, buns, bagels, pita, tortilla, cereal, crackers, popcorn, waffles, pancakes, grits, cornmeal, oats, rice, baked beans, corn, potatoes, sweet potatoes (yams), peas, beans, biscuits, chow mein noodles, french fries
Other Carbohydrate (equal to 1 starch or 1 fruit or 1 milk)	Carbohydrate, 15 grams	60 calories	Varies	cake, cookies, doughnuts, fruit snacks, fruit spreads, hummus, ice cream, chocolate milk, jam, jelly, pies, potato chips, syrup, sugar, tortilla chips, frozen yogurt, honey, sorbet, sherbet, canned spaghetti sauce, canned pasta sauce
Fruit	Carbohydrate, 15 grams	60 calories	1 sm/med whole; 1/2 cup canned or juice;	fresh, dried, or canned apples, apricots, bananas, berries, cherries, cantaloupe, figs, grapes, raisins, grapefruit,

Food Exchange Category	Food Type Energy Sources	Energy (Calorie) Value	Amounts/ Serving Sizes	Sample Foods
	Carbohydrate, 15 grams	25 calories	1/4 cup dried	kiwi, melon, mangos, papaya, oranges, watermelon, peaches, pears; fruit juices
Vegetable	Carbohydrate, 5 grams Protein, 2 grams		1 cup raw, 1/2 cup cooked	fresh or canned asparagus, beets, green beans, wax beans, artichokes, broccoli, brussels sprouts, beets, cabbage, sauerkraut, carrots, cauliflower, celery, cucumbers, greens, kohlrabi, onions, okra, salad greens, lettuce, mushrooms, peppers, radishes, spinach, tomatoes, turnips, zucchini; tomato sauce, vegetable juices
Milk, Nonfat & Lowfat	Carbohydrate, 12 grams Protein, 8 grams Fat, 3 grams or less	90 calories	1 cup	nonfat milk, nonfat buttermilk, 1% milk, plain nonfat yogurt, nonfat yogurt with fruit & nonsugar sweetener
Milk, Reduced Fat	Carbohydrate, 12 grams Protein, 8 grams Fat, 5 grams	120 calories	1 cup	2% milk, plain lowfat yogurt, lowfat yogurt with fruit & nonsugar sweetener; sweet acidophilus milk
Milk, Whole	Carbohydrate, 12 grams Protein, 8 grams Fat, 8 grams	150 calories	1 cup	whole milk, canned evaporated whole milk, goat's milk
Meat & Meat Substitutes, Very Lean	Protein, 7 grams Fat, 1 gram or less	35 calories	1 ounce or 1/2 cup	skinless white meat turkey, chicken, duck, pheasant; fresh or canned (in water) white-fleshed fish; lowfat lunch meats and cheeses; crab, clams, shrimp, scallos,

(continued)

Food Exchange Category	Food Type Energy Sources	Energy (Calorie) Value	Amounts/ Serving Sizes	Sample Foods
(Meat & Meat Substitutes, Very Lean contined)				lobster, imitation shellfish products; cooked beans and lentils
Meat & Meat Substitutes, Lean	Protein, 7 grams Fat, 3 grams	55 calories	1 ounce or 1/2 cup	USDA select or choice lean beef cuts with all visible fat trimmed (round, sirloin, flank steak; tenderloin; rib, chuck, rump roast; T-bone, porter- house, cubed steak; ground round); lean pork, ham, Canadian bacon; lamb; skinless dark meat chicken, turkey, duck, goose; herring, oysters, salmon, catfish, sardines, tuna canned in oil, cottage cheese, parmesan cheese, lowfat hotdogs, low- fat cheese, lowfat processed lunch meats
Meat & Meat Substitutes, Medium-Fat	Protein, 7 grams Fat, 5 grams	75 calories	1 ounce or 1/2 cup	other beef grades and cuts (ground beef, corned beef, ribs, prime rib); pork top loin, chops, cutlets; ground or roast lamb; veal; chicken dark meat with skin; fried chicken with skin; ground turkey or chicken; fried fish; eggs; tofu; tempeh; soy milk; feta, mozzarella, ricotta, cheese
Meat & Meat Substitutes, High-Fat	Protein, 7 grams Fat, 8 grams	100 calories	1 ounce or 1/2 cup	pork spareribs and sausage; ground pork; American, ched- dar, Monterey Jack, Swiss cheese; processed sandwich meats; sausage; chicken and turkey hot dogs; bacon; count also as 1 fat exchange: beef, pork, combination hotdogs; peanut butter made with unsaturated fat

Food Exchange Category	Food Type Energy Sources	Energy (Calorie) Value	Amounts/ Serving Sizes	Sample Foods
Fat	Fat, 5 grams	45 calories	1 tsp to 2 tbsp	oils, avocados, olives, almonds, cashews, peanuts, Brazil nuts, pecans, peanut butter, butter, mayonnaise, walnuts, salad dressing, coconut, fatback, salt pork, cream, half & half, sour cream, cream cheese, shortening, lard, bacon grease, sesame seeds, pumpkin seeds, sunflower seeds, chitterlings
Free Foods	n/a	20 calories or less	n/a	cooking spray, broth, ketchup, horseradish, lemon juice, lime juice, mustard, pickles, soy sauce, taco sauce, salsa, vinegar, garlic, herbs, spices, hot sauce, Worcestershire sauce, flavoring, pimento, sugar-free hard candy, sugar substitutes, fat-free cream cheese, nondairy creamer, fat-free or reduced fat sour cream, fat-free salad dressing, fat-free or reduced fat mayonnaise dressing, fat-free or reduced-fat margarine, coffee, tea, club soda, mineral water, unsweetened cocoa powder, sugar-free soft drinks

Some food exchange values differ *within* a particular food group. This is because many foods contain different combinations of food types in their makeup: that is, they are a blend of fat, protein, and/or carbohydrate. Let's take a look at meat to show you what we mean. We know that fat has more calories per ounce than protein. Meat contains both fat and protein; the value of one food exchange for meat changes according to the meat's fat component. Meat with a low percentage of fat has a lower calorie value, per exchange, than meat with a high percentage of fat does. One ounce of lean meat has fewer calories (50 calories) than one ounce of high-fat meat (100 calories).

Meats and Meat Substitutes	Very Lean	Lean	Medium-Fat	High-Fat
Protein	7 grams	7 grams	7 grams	7 grams
Fat	1 gram or less	3 grams	5 grams	8 grams
Calories	35	55	75	100

Once you know your daily calorie target, you choose each day's foods by the food exchange value that you want to include in each meal. Remember that a food exchange often differs from a serving size. One meat exchange = 1 ounce of meat; one serving of meat = 3 ounces = three meat exchanges. Here are the Menu for Life Meal Planner food exchanges in a table, for easy reference:

	1,800-Calorie Menu	2,100-Calorie Menu	2,400-Calorie Menu
Breakfast	3 starch/bread	3 starch/bread	3 starch/bread
	1 meat	2 meat	3 meat
	1 fruit	1 fruit	1 fruit
	1 milk	1 milk	1 milk
	2 fat	2 fat	free foods
	free foods	free foods	
AM Snack	1 fruit	1 fruit	1 fruit
Lunch	2 starch/bread	3 starch/bread	4 starch/bread
	2 meat	3 meat	4 meat
	2 vegetable	2 vegetable	2 vegetable
	2 fat	2 fat	2 fat
	1 fruit	1 fruit	1 fruit
	free foods	free foods	free foods
PM Snack	1 meat	1 starch/bread	1 starch/bread
	1 milk	1 meat	1 meat
	2 fruit	1 milk	1 milk
	2 starch/bread	1 fruit	1 fruit
Dinner	3 starch/bread	4 starch/bread	5 starch/bread
	3 meat	3 meat	3 meat
	2 vegetables	3 vegetables	4 vegetables
	2 fat	3 fat	3 fat
	1 fruit	1 fruit	1 fruit
	free foods	free foods	free foods

Each of the elements of the Menu for Life nutritional synergy—food type, food group, and food exchanges—gives you a different way to view and think about the foods you eat and how they fit into a plan for eating that balances your body's energy and nutritional needs with your personal tastes.

- **Food type**—lets you choose foods that supply your body with a healthy balance of the energy sources it needs
- **Food group**—gives you variety in choosing foods that give you the vitamins, minerals, and other nutrients that your body needs to meet the RDAs for healthy, balanced nutrition
- **Food exchanges**—let you incorporate a food value (calorie content) as you make choices about what, and how much food, you eat

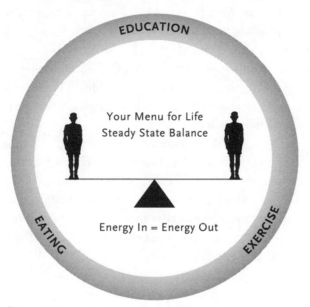

The Three Es of Energy Balance

We know it might take some time, some trial and error, for you to get used to thinking about food and meal planning the Menu for Life way, to put this new knowledge about the food you eat to work as you build your personalized Meal Planners. Have patience. Know that *you can*. Like anything else you put your mind and heart to, with practice meal planning will become second nature to you—the food types, food groups, and food exchanges will become a part of who you are. And always remember, this Menu for Life synergy works *for* you. Eating in this way allows you to *participate.* You leave the reactive, passive mode behind. This means taking responsibility, but it also means that *you choose.* No longer do you follow this diet or that diet. Because you have become educated about eating and exercise, you know how your body functions and what it needs. You create the balance that produces your Menu for Life synergy of health and well-being.

YOUR FOOD JOURNAL

Your food journal helps you to accomplish your first step in restoring your Energy In/Energy Out balance: to stop gaining weight. It helps you to do that by establishing where you are, *right now,* in terms of *what* and *how much* you eat. For the next two weeks, we want you to write down *everything* you eat and drink, and how much of it. *Everything that crosses your lips.*

To make this work, your food journal *must* be truthful; this is the only way you can determine how you need to reshape your eating habits so you can move toward creating your Menu for Life Meal Planner. For these two weeks, eat as you normally do—don't make any changes! Just keep track of what and how much you eat.

Keeping up with your food journal means more than taking five minutes right before you go to bed at night to scribble something down (or doing it a couple of days after the fact when you finally get a few spare moments to sit down and try remembering). What you need to do is get a small notebook, one you can carry with you everywhere you go, that fits easily in your pocket or your purse. At the top of each page in your notebook, write these headings:

- Food
- Drink
- How Much
- When/Where

Every time you put something in your mouth, write it in your notebook. If you order two fast-food meals and eat them for lunch, write it down. If you drink two large glasses of milk with breakfast, write it down. Don't worry that you don't know how much the glass holds. Describe the glass in such a way that you know what it is; later you can measure to see how much the glass holds. *Be absolutely honest.* Write down the times that you eat and drink too, so you can develop a sense of your eating patterns. Do you eat mostly at meals, mostly in between meals, or all the time? If you find yourself eating because you are under stress, or for some other emotional reason, put an asterisk beside that entry, or mark it with a colored pen or highlighter.

We ask you to do this so you can determine how and where you will need to focus on your eating. We do not mean to embarrass you; we mean to open your eyes! Change comes from the inside out. When you know what you are eating, how you are eating, and why you are eating, then you can develop the skills to change unhealthy eating into a healthful Menu for Life.

Donna has created what a page in a food journal might look like (see page 188), with entries from someone who eats about 2,400 calories a day.

When your two weeks of food journaling are up, take a good look at your data. If there are a lot of asterisks or highlights, you know that emotional eating is a factor for you. If you are eating at erratic times and places (or just all the time, everywhere!), you know that setting boundaries on where and when you eat will help you control your eating.

The next step, and this will take some figuring, is to look at what you are eating and how much. Choose a representative day from the two weeks of entries in your notebook, one you feel is typical of what and how much you eat. Compare what you wrote to the entries in Donna's sample 2,400-calorie day. Do you eat more or less food? You don't have to be a dietitian or measure the quantities and calorie values to know whether you are eating too much! If you are eating more food in a day than the amount of food in Donna's sample, your Energy In is too high and you need to work on that.

Now, try to fit what you ate into one of the three food types: fat, protein, and carbohydrate. Because most foods contain two or three of these energy sources, choose the food type that is the predominant one. (See page 180 for a list.) For example, vegetables are mostly carbohydrate and some protein, but no fat; so, list vegetables as carbohydrates. Next, identify which of the six food groups each item of food belongs to. We filled in one example from Donna's sample food journal to get you started. Finish the chart with foods from *your* food journal.

How many of your foods fit easily into either category: food type or food group? How much of what you eat and drink defies classification? Pack-

FOOD	DRINK	HOW MUCH	WHEN/WHERE
Bagel w/lowfat, fruit-flavored cream cheese		One whole bagel, cream cheese spread generously to cover both sides	7 a.m., kitchen
	Coffee w/fat-free creamer	12-ounce cup	7 a.m., kitchen
Chocolate chip cookies*		3	8:30 a.m.—a.m. break, in the car
	Coffee, black	12-ounce mug	10 a.m. meeting, office
Ham and Swiss on rye w/mayo, Dijon mustard, lettuce, tomato, pickle		Whole sandwich	11:30 a.m.—lunch, in the break room
	Diet root beer	12-ounce bottle	11:30 a.m.—lunch
Pretzels		5-ounce bag	11:30 a.m.—lunch
	Water	1-liter bottle	1 p.m., at desk
Baggie of fresh cherries		20–30 cherries	2:30 p.m., at desk
Banana		1	4 p.m., on the run
Chicken teriyaki w/steamed rice and steamed broccoli		Takeout dinner	6:30 p.m., in the living room in front of the TV
	Diet iced tea, bottled	16 ounces	6:30 p.m., all over the house
Lowfat frozen yogurt		1/2 cup	6:50 p.m., standing at the kitchen counter

*Eaten for an emotional reason.

FOOD OR DRINK	PRIMARY FOOD TYPE	PRIMARY FOOD GROUP
Broccoli	Carbohydrate	Vegetable

aged foods, processed foods, fast foods, and snack foods are hard to categorize because they *don't* fit. Most foods that don't fit are blends of fat and carbohydrate, and belong in the fats and sweets food group! These foods *do not* meet nutritional and health needs, and they *cannot* provide balanced energy for your body.

In laying out your Menu for Life Meal Planner, we will work with you on achieving daily calorie targets while rebalancing the proportion of fat, protein, and carbohydrate to give you the optimal benefits of 25 percent fat, 12 to 15 percent protein, and 55 to 60 percent carbohydrate. That proportion of food types at the daily number of calories you need each day allows you to use the food exchanges to select the foods you desire.

WEEKLY MEAL PLANNER

We've created Menu for Life Meal Planners with suggested food exchanges for three daily calorie targets: 1,800, 2,100, and 2,400 calories a day. Photocopy the meal planners as much as you like and use them to plan your week's meals and menus. If you are eating more than the 2,400 calorie target, work toward the target by reducing the amount of calories you take in by about 500 to 1,000 calories a day. Eating in this way, you have enough food, and the right kinds of food, to leave you feeling satisfied and nourished. This is enough of a drop for you to lose one to two pounds a week; losing weight any faster than one to two pounds a week is unhealthy for you, as we've discussed before.

Donna has given you an example by creating sample meals for two consecutive days, Tuesday and Wednesday, using the 2,400-calorie target Menu for Life Meal Planner. Examine the samples to familiarize yourself with the process of using food types, food groups, and food exchanges to design your own daily menus that provide the nutrients you need and the tastes you love.

In the chart that follows Donna also breaks out the process she used for selecting the foods for each meal, the serving size or amount of each food, and the food exchange values. Donna's recipes for the menu items are in bold type, and can be found in the recipe section of this book. Even though 2,400 calories might not sound like much to you now, this menu includes quite a lot of food. You may find, to your surprise, this is all the food you need and *want* to eat.

Here are a few planning pointers to notice:

- Choose entrees for the week that cover a range of meat, poultry, fish, or vegetarian alternatives to create variety in your meals—and in your leftovers! As you'll see, we use leftovers from Tuesday's dinner entree to make a salad for lunch on Wednesday, and from Tuesday's side dish salad for Wednesday's PM Snack.
- For some meals, there are unused food exchanges. You can use these exchanges as substitutes in another meal in the day or leave them unused. You don't have to use *all* of the food exchanges just because they are available!
- We use cauliflower florets for lunch on Tuesday and again in the vegetable side dish for dinner Wednesday.
- You can use food exchanges to create variety and menus that you enjoy. If you don't like cottage cheese for breakfast, for example, you can substitute three meat exchanges instead, such as turkey bacon. Or, you can pull a fat exchange from another meal where you haven't used it, such as lunch Tuesday in our example, and substitute a three-ounce serving of pork sausage as one highfat meat exchange.
- For foods such as crackers, check the package label for the serving size. (And always look for low sodium content in snack foods!)
- Alcohol used in cooking, such as the optional rum in the Broiled Citrus Swordfish, evaporates during the cooking process. Because it is the alcohol that accounts for the calories, once the alcohol evaporates the beverage used for cooking is a free food exchange. Alcohol consumed as a beverage, however, *does* have caloric content. If you do decide to have a glass of wine, a cocktail, or a beer, you must consider its caloric value in calculating your daily calories. Alcohol's caloric value is seven calories per gram or fluid ounce. Limiting alcohol consumption is a wise choice for a Menu for Life.
- With recipes and combinations, we show you the primary ingredients so you can see where the food exchanges come from. When you follow your own recipes or make combinations such as salads and sandwiches, determine their food exchanges in the same way, from the main ingredients.
- Drink water whenever you can, with your meals and throughout the day.

2,400 CALORIES A DAY	MEAL (FOODS)	SERVING SIZE/AMOUNT	FOOD EXCHANGES
Tuesday Breakfast	**Creamy Cornbread Muffin**	3 ounces	3 starch/bread
3 starch/bread	Lowfat cottage cheese	3/4 cup	3 meat
3 meat	Sliced fresh peaches	1/2 cup	1 fruit
1 fruit	Nonfat or 1% milk	1 cup	1 milk
1 milk	Coffee or tea	1 cup	free
free foods	Nondairy, nonfat creamer	to taste	free
	Non-sugar sweetener	to taste	free
Tuesday AM Snack	Sliced strawberries	3/4 cup	1 fruit
1 fruit	Non-sugar sweetener	to taste	free
Tuesday Lunch	Turkey sandwich:		
4 starch/bread	whole wheat bread	2 slices	2 starch/bread
4 meat	sliced deli turkey	3 ounces	3 meat
2 vegetable	lowfat mayonnaise	1 tablespoon	1 fat
2 fat	Dijon mustard	1 teaspoon	free
1 fruit	Swiss cheese	1 slice (1 ounce)	1 meat
free foods	Romaine lettuce	3-4 leaves	1 vegetable
	Cauliflower florets (raw)	1/2 cup	1 vegetable
	Herb Garden Dip (Nonfat)	1 tablespoon	free
	Cantaloupe	1/4 medium melon	1 fruit
	Diet soda	12 ounces	free
Tuesday PM Snack	Whole wheat crackers	6-8 crackers (1 ounce)	1 starch/bread
1 starch/bread			
1 meat	Sliced cheddar cheese	1 ounce	1 meat (high fat)
1 milk	Apple	1 medium	1 fruit
1 fruit			
Tuesday Dinner	**Broiled Citrus Swordfish**	3 ounces fish	3 meat
5 starch/bread	**with Caribbean Chutney:**	1/8 cup chutney	free
3 meat	Swordfish steak		
4 vegetables	lime juice		
3 fat	pineapple juice		
1 fruit	grapefruit juice		
free foods	bell pepper		
	green onion		
	tomato		
	papaya		
	mango		
	seasonings		
	Better-Than-Fried Potatoes:		
	baking or sweet potatoes	1 potato	1 starch/bread

(continued)

2,400 Calories a Day	Meal (Foods)	Serving Size/Amount	Food Exchanges
(Tuesday Dinner continued)	butter-flavored nonstick spray		
	Steamed broccoli	1 cup	2 vegetable
	Mixed salad greens	1/2 cup	1 vegetable
	Fat-free salad dressing	1 tablespoon	free
	Bread sticks	2	1 starch/bread
	Nonfat or 1% Milk	1 cup	1 milk (carried over from p.m. Snack)
	Sweet-Tart Fruit Salad:		
	strawberries	1 cup	1 fruit
	blackberries or black raspberries		1 vegetable
	cantaloupe		
	honeydew melon		
	seedless oranges		
	salad greens		
	Chocolate Spice Cake with Dark Chocolate Glaze	1 slice (1/12th of cake)	2 fat, 2 other carbohydrate (exchange for 2 starch/bread)
Wednesday Breakfast 3 starch/bread 3 meat 1 fruit 1 milk free foods	Scrambled eggs (add onion and red bell pepper if desired)	2 eggs, 1/4 cup nonfat or 1% milk	2 meat, 1/2 milk
	Turkey bacon	3 slices	1 meat
	English muffin	1 whole (top and bottom)	2 starch/bread
	Lowfat margarine (on muffin)	1 tablespoon	1 fat
	Jelly or jam (on muffin)	1 tablespoon	1 other carbohydrate (exchange for 1 starch)
	Orange, fresh	1 medium	1 fruit
	Nonfat or 1% milk	1 cup	1 milk
	Coffee or tea	1 cup	free
	Nondairy, nonfat creamer	to taste	free
	Non-sugar sweetener	to taste	free
Wednesday AM Snack 1 fruit	Lowfat yogurt with fruit	1/2 cup	1 other carbohydrate (exchange for 1 fruit)

2,400 Calories a Day	Meal (Foods)	Serving Size/Amount	Food Exchanges
Wednesday Lunch	Citrus Swordfish Salad		
4 starch/bread	leftover swordfish from	3 ounces	3 meat
4 meat	Tuesday dinner		
2 vegetable	leftover Caribbean chutney	1 tablespoon	free
2 fat	salad greens	2 cups	2 vegetable
1 fruit	French bread, warmed in	2 slices (2 ounces)	2 starch/bread
free foods	oven		1 fat
	Lowfat margarine on bread	1 tablespoon	1 fruit
	if desired)		free
	Grapes	3 ounces	free
	Iced tea	12 ounces	
	Nonsugar sweetener in tea	to taste	
	if desired		
Wednesday PM Snack	Sweet-Tart Fruit Salad		
1 starch/bread	(leftover)	1/2 cup	1 fruit
1 meat	Popcorn (unbuttered)	3 cups	1 starch/bread
1 milk	Frozen yogurt, fat-free and	1/2 cup	1 other carbohy-
1 fruit	sugar-free		drate (exchange
			for 1 milk)
Wednesday Dinner	**Green Chile Chicken**	1 chicken breast,	3 meat
5 starch/bread	**Casserole:**	1/2 cup casserole	1 milk
3 meat	skinless, boneless chicken		1 starch/bread
4 vegetables	breast		1 fat
3 fat	lowfat chicken broth		1/2 vegetable
1 fruit	cornmeal		
free foods	margarine		
	nonfat buttermilk		
	green chiles		
	corn		
	seasonings		
	Long grain rice	1/2 cup	1 starch/bread
	Multigrain rolls	1 roll	
	Lowfat margarine on roll if	1 tablespoon	
	desired		
	Nutty Broccoli Toss:	1 cup	2 vegetable
	cauliflower		1 meat (exchange
	broccoli		for 1 fat)
	nuts		1 fat
	sunflower seeds		

(continued)

2,400 Calories a Day	Meal (Foods)	Serving Size/Amount	Food Exchanges
(Wednesday Dinner continued)	seasonings		
	Angel food cake with strawberries and lowfat whipped cream	1 slice (1/12th of cake)	2 other carbohydrates (exchange for 2 starch)
		1/2 cup strawberries	1 fruit
		1/4 cup lowfat whipped cream	1 other carbohydrate (exchange for 1 starch)

When you plan your meals and menus, here are some additional tips and strategies.

- Think about how the food will look when you serve it. Visual qualities such as color, shape, and texture make food look like it tastes good. (Too many brown foods, cubed foods, and cut up foods are dull—at least to Donna!) When you think food tastes good, you want to eat it—which is very important when these are foods that are very good for you. So go ahead, play with your food! Put foods together that you are used to seeing together and experiment with unfamiliar combinations. Changing the way your food looks changes the way you feel about eating it and encourages you to try new and different things.
- Plan your main dishes first, consider how many ingredients you will need to buy, what the cooking method is (roast, grill, broil, bake, steam)—you'll want to vary this from day to day—how long the meal will take to prepare, and whether you'll have enough for leftovers.
- Decide which vegetables you want to highlight as side dishes, in soups, stews, chili, or lasagna, or in salads. Choose a range of vegetables with different vitamin and mineral content. Always consider vegetables that are in season.
- Choose fresh fruits whenever you can
- When planning a lunch salad, consider making the salad heartier than the evening meal. Then, choose a light supper alternative.
- Avoid repetition in flavors and food choices. Variety is the spice of life—and keeps your menus interesting and your family and guests coming back for more!
- Avoid processed foods and snacks.

• Stay with it. Every now and then you'll have an idea that doesn't quite work out the way you intend. So what? The more weekly menus you plan, the better you'll get at doing it. You'll learn to create cost-effective, time-effective, nutrition-boosting meals that hit the calorie targets and satisfy your tastes, time, and budget.

Here is how Donna's two days' worth of sample meals looks on the Weekly Meal Planner:

WEEKLY MEAL PLANNER 2,400

	BREAKFAST	AM SNACK	LUNCH	PM SNACK	DINNER
2,400 Calories a Day	3 starch/bread 3 meat 1 fruit 1 milk free foods	1 fruit	4 starch/bread 4 meat 2 vegetable 2 fat 1 fruit free foods	1 starch/bread 1 meat 1 milk 1 fruit	5 starch/bread 3 meat 4 vegetables 3 fat 1 fruit free foods
Tuesday	Creamy Corn- bread Muffin Lowfat cottage cheese Sliced fresh peaches Nonfat or 1% milk Coffee or tea Nondairy, nonfat creamer Non-sugar sweetener	Sliced strawber- ries Non-sugar sweetener	Turkey sandwich Cauliflower florets (raw) Herb Garden Dip (Nonfat) Cantaloupe Diet soda	Whole wheat crackers Sliced cheddar cheese Apple	Broiled Citrus Swordfish with Caribbean Chutney Better-than-Fried Potatoes Steamed broccoli Mixed salad greens Fat-free salad dressing Bread sticks Nonfat or 1% milk Sweet-Tart Fruit Salad Chocolate Spice Cake with Dark Chocolate Glaze

(continued)

WEEKLY MEAL PLANNER 2,400

	Breakfast	am Snack	Lunch	pm Snack	Dinner
Wednesday	Scrambled eggs (add onion and red bell pepper if desired) Turkey bacon English muffin Lowfat margarine (on muffin) Jelly or jam (on muffin) Orange, fresh Nonfat or 1% milk Coffee or tea Nondairy, nonfat creamer Nonsugar sweetener	Lowfat yogurt with fruit	Citrus Swordfish salad (using leftovers) French bread Lowfat margarine on bread if desired Grapes Iced tea Nonsugar sweetener in tea if desired	Sweet-Tart Fruit Salad (leftover) Popcorn (unbuttered) Frozen yogurt, fat-free and sugar-free	Green Chile Chicken Casserole Long grain rice Multigrain rolls Lowfat margarine on roll if desired Nutty Broccoli Toss Angel food cake w/strawberries and lowfat whipped cream

After you complete your Weekly Meal Planner, make a shopping list. (We created a blank shopping list form you can photocopy as much as you like.) Do this when the meals you have planned are still fresh in your mind. Then take your list to the grocery store, where it will be both your *guide* and your *shield*. Because your shopping list contains the ingredients for the meals you intend to prepare for the week, it will guide you to make the right food choices in the grocery store. Your shopping list will also shield you against impulse purchases, especially when you walk the gauntlet of "specials" and promotions when you first enter the store. When you feel tempted to reach out for one of those bargains, look at your list. Unless you see that item written there, pass. There is no impulse buy or bargain that is worth the price of your health!

Okay, so we've shown you how to use food types, food groups, and food exchanges to plan healthful weekly meals. Now it is your turn to use the Meal Planners to create *your* family's Menu for Life. Get planning! Start with your main dishes, take your time, think it through, and plan carefully. Take a look at Donna's recipes and see what whets your appetite. When your Menu for Life Weekly Meal Planner and Shopping List are ready, let's go shopping with Donna.

WEEKLY MEAL PLANNER 2,400

	Breakfast	am Snack	Lunch	pm Snack	Dinner
2,400 Calories a Day	3 starch/bread 3 meat 1 fruit 1 milk free foods	1 fruit	4 starch/bread 4 meat 2 vegetable 2 fat 1 fruit free foods	1 starch/bread 1 meat 1 milk 1 fruit	5 starch/bread 3 meat 4 vegetables 3 fat 1 fruit free foods

Monday

Tuesday

Wednesday

Thursday

Friday

Saturday

Sunday

WEEKLY MEAL PLANNER 2,100

	Breakfast	am Snack	Lunch	pm Snack	Dinner
2,100 **Calories** **a Day**	3 starch/bread	1 fruit	3 starch/bread	1 starch/bread	4 starch/bread
	2 meat		3 meat	1 meat	3 meat
	1 fruit		2 vegetable	1 milk	3 vegetables
	1 milk		2 fat	1 fruit	3 fat
	2 fat		1 fruit		1 fruit
	free foods		free foods		free foods

Monday

Tuesday

Wednesday

Thursday

Friday

Saturday

Sunday

WEEKLY MEAL PLANNER 1,800

	BREAKFAST	AM SNACK	LUNCH	PM SNACK	DINNER
1,800 CALORIES A DAY	3 starch/bread 1 meat 1 fruit 1 milk 2 fat free foods	1 fruit	2 starch/bread 2 meat 2 vegetable 2 fat 1 fruit free foods	2 starch/bread 1 meat 1 milk 2 fruit	3 starch/bread 3 meat 2 vegetables 2 fat 1 fruit free foods

Monday

Tuesday

Wednesday

Thursday

Friday

Saturday

Sunday

WEEKLY SHOPPING LIST

Meat, Poultry, Fish, Dried Beans, Eggs	Dairy (Milk, Cheese, Yogurt)	Breads & Grains	Vegetables	Fruits	Spices & Seasonings

Part Four

~~~~~

Have Your Cake and Eat It Too!

10

~~~~~~~

Shopping with Donna:
Going for Groceries

*T*hey tempt you, right from the start. There you are, standing in the entrance of your favorite grocery store, and the first sight that greets you when you walk through the store's automatic doors is every shopper's favorite four-letter word: SALE! Bargains, specials, deals presented in enticing front-of-the-store displays you can't miss because they are right there, placed physically between you and the rest of the store. Usually these displays are for snack or other convenience foods, items that may be a little pricey normally, holiday or seasonal items, or new items a manufacturer wants you to try. *Today only! Buy two, get one free. Buy one, get the second one for half-price. Limit five per customer.* And when the store is feeling especially generous, *buy one and get one free.* How can you ignore these extraordinary savings? Say it again, "I can." And *keep on walking.*

Unless there is a fabulous special on toilet tissue—because you can never have too much toilet tissue—it is unlikely there is any food item here that you need. Hold onto your Menu for Life shopping list and feel confident. *You* are in control of how you spend your money in the store, what you buy, and which products are true bargains for you. You are a Menu for Life food artist, and you are on a mission to create healthful meals you plan each week. Marketing ploys no longer have the power to sway you from your path to a beautiful life. You know how and where to find the best value for your money *and* for your health—and that may not be where the store is begging you to spend your money. You shop to buy what you need, to buy what's on your list, *to buy what you want*, not what the store wants you to buy.

It is no accident that the meat department, produce section, and dairy case are all in the *back* of every grocery store. Meat, produce, and dairy are the items you purchase all the time, and if they were easy for you to get to, you would buy simply what you *need* and be out of the store. The store's mission is to get you to *spend your money*, as much of it as possible, as much of it as they can get you to part with. So there are displays and specials and bargains at the front of the store, and once in the store, there are aisles filled with temptations to appeal to the part of you that buys on impulse. The business of selling to you, of getting you to buy certain products and more products, is highly competitive. Manufacturers want your dollars, so they pay big money to buy premium shelf space, space extensive consumer research tells them is most effective for catching your attention, space you can see and reach without effort.

DONNA RANDALL

"Okay, so who is in charge here? *You are.* As a Menu for Life shopper, you have your eyes wide open and you see through the fancy packaging, the advertising claims, and the special offers that are doing more of a favor for the store than for you—and I'm talking about both your health and your wallet!

"You know, a lot of people are into yoga and meditation these days as ways to reduce stress and get exercise with these practices and you hear a lot about the concept of mindfulness—mindful walking, for example, or mindful meditative breathing. To be mindful means to be fully aware of what it is that you are doing, in the present moment, and to do it with the joy and commitment of your whole being. So what about *mindful eating?* When you plan your meals with the Menu for Life meal planner and do your shopping list and cook healthful meals for your family at home, you are practicing mindful eating. Mindful eating is smart, conscious, aware eating. Go into the grocery store with your Menu for Life shopping list. Know that you are acting mindfully about what, when, where, why, and how you are eating. Take charge. You *can!*"

DR. RANDALL

"People love to shop with Donna. The grocery store can be a tough challenge for many people, maybe for you too. You go in with the best intentions, but get waylaid or confused about how to do your shopping, what to buy that is healthy to eat, how to read food labels, and generally make good choices between different products and kinds of foods. Donna shows you how to shop in accordance with the Menu for Life program. Shopping may take a new kind of effort and concentration, but with Donna's guidance it is easy, fun, and well worth it. You'll find your investment pays off in ways you may not initially expect. You'll see improvements ranging from greater efficiency and use of your time when shopping, to financial savings overall in shopping and buying wisely, to the best benefit of all—the immeasurable benefit of health and well-being that comes with eating healthfully the Menu for Life way. So enjoy shopping with Donna. Indulge your passion for food in a way that is creative and healthful for you!"

Every grocery store you go into has its unique layout to draw you in and get you to spend more money than you planned—to buy items not on your Menu for Life shopping list. Stores know, for example, that you want to go to the bakery section to buy all of your baked goods . . . so they make you go to several locations in the store to find everything you need. Packaged, brand-name breads and rolls are in one place, while the fresh-baked breads are in another. Cereals, of course, are in an aisle of their own. So even following your Menu for Life shopping list becomes an odyssey that takes you up and down every aisle, into every department of the grocery store— because that's what store owners want. Store owners want you to walk every aisle and eyeball every display. They are counting on the full-color photographs of food on the packaging to literally get your mouth watering so you'll reach out and grab that box or bag and take it home. Manufacturers want you to buy your way out of the store!

You, as a Menu for Life shopper, however, are no easy marketing target. Armed with your shopping list, you know what you need and want to prepare healthful weekly meals for yourself and your family before you set one foot in the store. Shopping list in hand, you will travel from location to location within the store, and that will be okay, because you will stay with your shopping list, and it will guide you to wise purchasing decisions and protect you from falling victim to marketing ploys and false bargains.

Read and Compare Product Labels and Packages

When you stand in the grocery store, all the choices and options can be overwhelming. So it is time for you to put into practice what you learned in Chapter 8 about reading and comparing food labels. Do you have a favorite brand of an item that is on your Menu for Life shopping list? Start with that brand and read the label. Notice:

- How much is a serving size?
- How many servings are in the container?
- How many total calories does one serving deliver?
- What nutrients do the product provide, and how much of each one?

Think about how you usually use or eat this product. Do you *really* consume just one serving? *Be honest with yourself.* If one serving size of a package of cookies is one cookie but you know you always eat three cookies, can you afford the Energy In cost of three cookies? If a box of frozen waffles says it contains four servings and you usually prepare and eat half the box yourself, then you have to double all of the numbers to get your Energy In value for this product. *Check the numbers.* You need to multiply all the information on the food label to correspond to the actual serving size you intend to eat. Doing this prevents you from being duped into perceiving products as if they are one serving when, in fact, the package or can holds so much more than that, and so many more calories, fat, or sodium than you may see at first glance. A 20-ounce beverage bottle is a perfect example. We are conditioned to believe this bottle is appropriate to consume in one serving, when, typically, a 20-ounce beverage holds 2 to 2 1/2 servings of that beverage. Reading labels in this way helps you to relate serving sizes to appropriate portion sizes and helps you maintain accurate portion control.

Cooking sprays are another good example of how closely you must read food labels. Cooking sprays contain cooking oil, usually canola oil, in an aerosol suspension. But a serving size delivers so little oil that the label can claim the product is fat-free—and it is, if you use no more than the label's stated serving size of a spray: *one-third of a second*! How do you measure that? At best you are likely to get a one-second burst, which is three times as much and delivers seven grams of fat. A three-second burst gives you 21 grams of fat and 189 calories—this from a "fat-free" product!

You cannot rely on advertising claims—fat-free, reduced sodium, sugar-free, light—to give you real-world information about *any* product's true nutritional value. Even though manufacturers sometimes go to great lengths to craft label language that favors their products, in the end it's the numbers on the food labels that tell the true story. So look at more than the words. Do the numbers.

Meat, Poultry, Fish, Dried Beans, Eggs

In the meat department, you want to look for the leanest meats your store offers. You say these leaner cuts are too expensive? Know that leaner is really *cheaper*. When you buy pork chops, half of what you are buying is fat and bone. Why pay for something you are just going to throw away? Buy the pork loin. If you feel that you must have ground beef, buy the leanest blend—usually less than 10 percent fat and when you cook it, use one of those pans with ridges specially designed to allow you to pour the fat away. If you usually buy a cut of meat like a chuck roast, which is marbled with fat, consider that you are *paying* for all that fat—at the cash register and with your health when your doctor tells you that you have high blood cholesterol. A round steak is lower in fat. And tough, you may say. But you can take an eye of a round and make it just as tender as any cut of beef you've ever eaten. Just rub it with a little marinade, cut slits in it, and stick garlic inside. Try the recipe for Marinated Beef Strips with Orange Brandy Sauce in the recipe section of this book—you'll see!

Also consider substituting chicken, fish, or turkey for beef, all of which contain lower amounts of fat. When buying turkey or chicken, you want to read your labels to look for added ingredients. Avoid whole birds that have fat in the form of butter or butter flavoring added to them. Opt instead for the low-fat breasts. Buy them skinless if the price is right, or remove the skin when you prepare them for cooking or freezing. For people who have to have the skin taste or texture, buy the chicken thighs; you can remove the thickest part of the skin and leave a little bit there to get that taste and texture you want. If you are going to cook a whole bird, say for a holiday meal, buy a small one. Remember that a serving size of meat is four ounces uncooked to produce three ounces cooked, and you want to buy only what you plan to cook and eat, so calculate how many people your recipe serves and buy a bird that holds only that much meat.

What about those "meal kits" and prepared meat products you can buy? Beef Wellington or Chicken Cordon Bleu straight in the oven! But what *kind* of meal are you really getting? Read the labels! Many of these products are quite high in fat and have too much added salt—convenience at a cost. You are better off preparing your meals at home from ingredients that you choose, knowing exactly what you are getting and knowing that you are getting the best. If you want deli meats for your sandwiches, that's fine. Most have nutritional information on the deli packaging and you can ask the deli counterperson to show you the food label if you have questions. The labels will reveal any added ingredients or high-fat or sodium content.

Fish is an excellent low-fat, high-protein choice. In general white, light fish will have less fat than fish that is of a dark color and firm flesh. Even fish varieties that are higher in fat, such as salmon, usually contain omega 3 fatty acids, a beneficial lipid that helps your cardiovascular system. Try to eat fish at least once a week. Choose fresh fish from a reputable grocer or fish market over frozen fish if you can. Fish should be prepared and eaten promptly—the same day you buy it is best. Stay away from pre-breaded fish products as they are likely to be higher in fat and sodium content. Cook your fish just about any way you want it—except for frying! Bake, broil, poach, grill, microwave. Try the Broiled Citrus Swordfish with Caribbean Chutney recipe in this book.

When buying any kind of meat, you want to divide it into appropriate portion sizes *before* freezing it at home. (Unless, of course, you are buying a whole bird, as we discussed above.) If you buy an eight-ounce steak you are planning to freeze to eat later in the week, make sure you cut it in half before you freeze it. This way it will be in individual serving portions, and you won't be tempted to cook and eat the whole steak. You can season your meat at this stage too, using whatever spices you like—but no added sodium. Sodium will draw moisture from the meat before it freezes, which will affect the meat's texture and tenderness. Pre-seasoning with flavorful seasonings other than sodium, however, can save a step in the cooking; all you have to do when you are ready to cook is defrost the meat and pop it on the grill, on top of the stove, or into the oven.

The same is true for economy size packages of meat. Economy packaging of meat can save you quite a lot of money but you have to be smart about how you use and freeze this meat. As soon as you get home, take that economy size package and break it out into single serving sizes. Season the meat at this time, as you desire. Separate enough meat out for one complete meal as called for by an individual recipe, then freeze the rest in individual packages. No matter how low the price, a three-pound package of chicken is no bargain if you have to defrost, cook, and eat the whole thing at one sitting! If you find it too tempting to have so much food available, avoid purchasing economy packs. Buy only the amount of meat you need for the recipe that is on your weekly meal planner.

Beans are another healthful and low-fat source of protein. Cooking with dried beans may seem like too much effort—but how hard is it to put a cup or two of beans in a bowl of water to soak or in a pot of boiling stock to soften? Not that hard! If you use canned beans in your recipes, be sure to rinse and drain them thoroughly, and always choose the brand with the lowest sodium content and no extra fats or other added ingredients. A nice quick side dish can be made by microwaving a potato for about 15 minutes until it is soft enough to mash. Mash in some red kidney beans, some minced garlic, and some fresh herbs, and enjoy it with a salad. For another bean alternative, try the Vegetarian Chili recipe in this book. Homemade chili is easy, fast, and very healthful. Canned chili? Leave it on the shelf.

Are eggs on your shopping list? When selecting eggs, chose those fortified with omega 3 fatty acids. You may also be able to find eggs laid by chickens raised to produce eggs that contain lesser amounts of saturated fats. These eggs may cost a little bit more, but if you like eggs, the benefit for your health is worth the slightly higher price. Of course, there are many egg substitute products available as well, and each one is a little bit different in the way it tastes and how it responds when you cook with it. Read the labels carefully to choose the product that is right for you.

DAIRY (MILK, CHEESE, YOGURT)

When it comes to milk and other dairy products, such as cheese and yogurt, the less fat the better. And again, labeling can be deceiving. Even *nonfat* milk contains some fat—about half a gram per one-cup serving. Do you drink just one cup, eight ounces? Many drinking glasses hold 12 or 16 ounces—so the lower the fat content of the milk, the better. Make sure you know what you are consuming. If you dislike the taste of nonfat milk, try 1 percent milk. If you are used to drinking whole milk, bump down to 2 percent milk first. Let your taste buds adjust—give them about two weeks. Soon enough, you will leave the high fat habit behind and develop the new habit (and the taste!) for lower fat foods. You may find that after a few months, nonfat milk tastes preferable. After you have gotten used to the taste of lower fat dairy products, the full fat versions will seem extraordinarily rich and heavy to your more sensitive taste buds. Some brands of reduced fat cheese and yogurts yield the same creamy taste and are not really that far from the texture and flavor of the higher fat varieties. The key is to read the labels and choose carefully.

You might say, okay I can do low-fat dairy but I must have my ice cream! Well, you can have your ice cream—but you need to eat less of it, less often. Sorbet is a wonderful low-fat alternative to ice cream, as is sherbet or ice milk. These frozen treats give you different tastes and textures you might like. Or try the Chai-Spiced Peach Mousse in the recipe section. Fresh fruit makes a wonderful and nutrient-dense alternative too, when you are craving some sweetness. If you absolutely must have that ice cream texture, try one of the gourmet lowfat frozen yogurts. You can even find delicious products now made with soy milk, a high-protein alternative.

BREADS AND GRAINS

Bread or rolls are probably on your shopping list. Here too you want to read the labels closely. Look at the sodium content per serving and make sure to check the serving size. You also want to look at the total number of calories per serving. Pick bread and rolls with low sodium and fewer calories and try to buy whole grains. Whole grain bread products have better nutrient density than white, and they give your body more of what you need and leave you feeling more satisfied. Is the brand of bread or rolls you prefer on sale? Buy what you need and plan to use for now and buy more to freeze. When freezing, make sure to break an economy package down into smaller portions that you can use up while the product is still fresh.

As with bread products, whole wheat grain or pasta products have more nutrient density. When buying boxed grain or pasta mixes, be careful to watch for added fat, sodium, or calories, and pay attention to the recommended serving size. It is often better to buy your grain or pasta without added flavors or seasonings and add your own when you cook at home. You can find terrific dried pasta, fresh pasta in the dairy case, or even fast-cooking lasagna noodles. If you love rice, invest in a rice cooker that makes cooking rice easy and predictable.

Products like breadcrumbs and croutons, because of their typically high fat and high sodium content, are better if you make them yourself at home. It is easy to make your own croutons. Use the bread crusts cut off of your children's sandwiches. Or use the stale end of a loaf of bread. Chop the bread into cubes and add some garlic and some herbs. If you want to, you can spritz the bread cubes with a non-fat cooking spray. Pop them in the oven and toast. Or you can buy plain breadcrumbs, without added seasonings, and mix in Italian seasonings or whatever you want to use. Then you have the flavors you like without the fat or sodium.

Breakfast cereals are quick and easy in the morning, but not so simple in the store. Your best bet is to stay away from the sweetened varieties. Your children and grandchildren may love sugary cereals, but you might as well feed them candy. Choose whole grain cereals and add a little honey at home or choose a lightly sweetened cereal. Some of the cereals that target children have 45 grams of sugar per serving! Some of the "healthy" cereals that target adults contain much more sugar and fat than you might expect, especially those with dried fruits and nuts added. Look too at the serving size. Remember the example from Chapter 8? One cereal might appear to have more nutrient density, but with a second, closer look you see that the serving size is less than another cereal. You have to compare closely.

Cakes, cookies, muffins, and items the store bakes and sells may not have the standard nutrition information labels you see on prepackaged baked goods. Often there is only a list of ingredients. When there is no nutritional information on the label, you can be sure the item is high in fat, high in sugar, and has little nutritional value. So that tray of cheese Danish—pass it by! If you crave these tastes, choose products that give you the nutritional information, ask the store to provide nutritional information for you, or, best yet, find a healthful recipe and make your own baked goodies.

Yes, you can still have your cake and eat it too! Plus the pride of baking it yourself. Forget box mixes and make your own from scratch with the same amount of effort. Try the recipe for Chocolate Spice Cake with Dark Chocolate Glaze in this book. When you make your own cake you know you are getting a delicious *and* healthful treat. Remember that in practicing your Menu for Life you are not trying to deprive yourself of the things that you love. The same goes for cookies, muffins, pies, and other delights. Check out the Creamy Cornbread Muffins recipe in this book or the Pear Tofu Cheesecake Amandine. Rich, satisfying, and healthful alternatives are right here at your fingertips.

VEGETABLES AND FRUITS

The produce section is the best place to shop for vegetables and fruits. Stand for a moment to admire the gorgeous, colorful variety. Vegetables and fruits are as good for you as they are to look at! When at all possible buy fresh fruits and vegetables—not just because they look better, but also because they have more nutrients than frozen or canned, and they contain no added fat or sodium.

When you plan your meals for the week, sit down with your store's weekly advertising circular to find out which fresh fruits and vegetables are going to be on sale. See if you can use the fresh sale items of the week in your weekly meal planner. (Check the circular for meat specials too.) Nowadays, you can buy fresh strawberries during just about any month of the year. But strawberries are in season in the summer, and that's when they are cheaper, fresher, and tastier. Oftentimes produce section specials feature seasonal offerings. So, you get a bargain and a fresher and tastier product too.

When you can't find the vegetables and fruits that you need in the produce section, your next stop is the freezer case. Frozen vegetables are the next best thing to fresh, as long as you buy *just* vegetables. Try vegetable mixes for variety, like a mix of peas and carrots or a mix of peas, carrots, corn, lima beans, and green beans. A variety of different vegetables mixed together gives you better nutrient density than one vegetable on its own. But avoid mixes that include butter-flavored sauce, cheese-flavored sauce, or other such variations. These "extras" add calories—and when you read the labels, you notice that few of these sauces actually contain any of the ingredients they are flavored to taste like. Some frozen vegetables also add sodium; this is not necessary, so choose products without sodium, monosodium glutamate (MSG), another common preservative, or other additives.

Frozen fruits are the next best thing to fresh fruits, but shop carefully. Often, manufacturers pack frozen fruits in sugar or syrup. Look for products that contain just the fruit. The same goes for canned fruits such as pears, peaches, pineapple, or fruit cocktail. Select ones that are packed in their own juices and not in heavy syrup. Fresh fruit, though, has much better nutrient density and will leave you feeling more satisfied than any type of fruit that comes out of a bag or a can. Add diced fresh fruit to yogurt for a creamy, flavorful dessert or to a salad for interesting texture and taste. You can also add a small amount of dried fruit for a similar effect, but be sure to look at the food label for dried fruits to check that they do not contain too many calories, extra sweeteners, or other unnecessary additives.

If the vegetable that you need is not available fresh or frozen, canned is an option. But canned is really the least desirable choice when it comes to vegetables. When vegetables undergo the canning process, they are subject to high heat that destroys a lot of their nutritional value. It also can destroy much of their taste! If you are going to buy vegetables in a can, be doubly sure they do not contain too much sodium. Canned goods in general can be very high in sodium. Many brands now offer low sodium options—and some stores even have small low sodium sections—so look for these. You also need to check the can's label for added fats and MSG.

Canned tomatoes are the one canned product worth buying, as cooking and processing tomatoes does not seem to greatly diminish their health-enhancing beneficial properties. Again, however, you want to read labels carefully for the sodium content and other additives in canned tomato products. If you plan, for example, to make your own barbecue sauce and you start off with a can of tomato sauce, know that you start with about 330 milligrams of sodium per serving. And that's before you begin cooking! Compare the sodium content for a can of crushed tomatoes which comes in at 150 milligrams of sodium per serving, or half of what is in the tomato sauce. Keep looking and you will see that tomato puree has an even lower sodium count at 30 milligrams per serving. So start your barbeque sauce right with a low sodium choice.

SALAD PRODUCE

Does your local supermarket carry pre-made salads in bags? Prepared salads can be great time savers, and they can add beneficial nutrients to your diet if you are a careful consumer. You will want to avoid salad kits that come with dressing and possibly croutons. These kits usually have high fat content and can have added sodium too. Instead look for prepared salad bags of precut fresh vegetables and mixed salad greens. Or buy bags of veggies, such as baby carrots or broccoli florets, and eat them raw with dips, or use them in the salads or entrees you've planned. Check out the Herb Garden Dip and the selection of salad dressing recipes in this book. If you buy pre-made dips and dressings, read the food labels carefully!

How about a salad of lettuces with grated vegetables such as carrots or radishes, or blends of various kinds of lettuces? There is more to salad than just iceberg! Do these other lettuces cost more? Sometimes they do. But consider that iceberg lettuce is all water. Why pay good money for that? Especially when you can buy other types of lettuces and greens—such as kale, young spinach, mustard greens, or chard—that are much more nutritive than iceberg lettuce and taste more satisfying too. Have you ever had a fresh green salad that you made yourself? Take Swiss chard, collard greens, spinach, romaine, and a selection of other lettuces. Chop them up for your salad. Add fresh tomatoes, red onion, pepper, a little bit of balsamic vinegar, and garlic. Every bite of your homemade salad will yield unique flavor sensations. Put in fresh herbs to create an exciting salad! Why not try some sprouts? Many stores now carry a variety of fresh vegetable sprouts such as mung, alfalfa, clover, radish, and sunflower. They have a fresh green taste, interesting texture, and lots of nutrient power.

What about convenient salad bars? Salad bars can be great time savers, especially on your lunch hour at work! But stay away from the high-fat, high-sodium temptations like prepared croutons, bacon pieces, avocado, nuts, seeds (sesame, sunflower, pumpkin), olives, and artichoke hearts. Hearts of palm and pickles don't have any fat to speak of, but they are very high in sodium. If any of these are your favorites, and you *must* have them, add sparingly—only enough to enjoy a taste of that flavor you love. Also consider that any salad that comes with dressing or mayonnaise already mixed in, such as potato salad or macaroni salad, will be high in fat.

So what *can* you put in your salad without worry? The choices are nearly endless when you use your imagination. Here are just a few suggestions to get you started.

Dairy Products	Nonfat cottage cheese, hard boiled egg, grated nonfat cheese, nonfat yogurt
Fruits	Apples, apricots, cranberries, dates, figs (fresh or dried), grapes, lemon, lime, mango, melon (cantaloupe, honeydew, Crenshaw), oranges, papaya, pears, persimmon, pineapple, plums, pomegranate, raisins, tangerines
Grains	Barley, Bulgur wheat, couscous, pasta, rice, quinoa
Herbs	Basil, chervil, chives, cilantro, dill, lemon verbena, lovage, marjoram, mint leaves, oregano, parsley, rosemary, tarragon, thyme, sage, sorrel
Legumes	Chickpeas (garbanzo beans), bean thread noodles, black-eyed peas, kidney beans, lentils, lima beans, navy beans, pinto beans, tofu, white beans
Meats	Beef, codfish, chicken, crabmeat, tuna
Spices	Anise seeds, caraway seeds, celery seed, cumin, ginger root, horseradish, mustard, pepper (black, red, white), poppy seeds
Vegetables	Alfalfa sprouts, arugala, asparagus, bean sprouts, beets (raw or boiled), broccoli, cabbage (green, red, Napa, Savoy, or bok choy), carrots, cauliflower, corn, cucumber (English, seedless, or kirbies), eggplant, endive, escarole, fennel, green beans, Jerusalem artichokes, jicama, kohlrabi, leeks, mushrooms, mustard greens, peas, peppers (raw, steamed, or roasted, sweet or hot), potatoes, radishes (red or white), radish sprouts, rutabaga, scallions, sea vegetables (arame, hijiki, dulse), shallots, snap peas in the pod, spinach, sunflower sprouts, turnips, watercress, zucchini

SPICES AND SEASONINGS

Having a nice variety of spices at home can make cooking your own meals a more flavorful, fun, and tasty experience, but some seasonings you may be accustomed to using, such as garlic salt, contain much more sodium than you want. Try garlic powder, or better, minced garlic instead. In addition, spice blends such as curry and Cajun or chili powders also contain high amounts of sodium. Read the label on boxes or jars of seasoning carefully! If your favorite seasoning does contain sodium, see if there is a no-sodium variety available. If not, why not buy all the spices in the mix and stir up a batch of your very own? This way you can tailor your spice experience and leave out the sodium altogether. Check the label of the mix, and remember that the ingredients always appear in the order of most to least. You might need to experiment to find the blend you want, but this can be fun, too.

Buying a lot of spices may seem expensive, but as you fill your spice rack you will find you won't need to buy an additional spice every time you try a new recipe. You will also discover what spices and spice combinations you love the most and come to rely on them as Menu for Life flavor standards. Try the homemade Cajun spice blend we include with the recipe for Oven-Fried Cajun Catfish.

THE TEMPTATIONS OF CONVENIENCE FOODS, CANNED FOODS, SNACK FOODS, AND OTHER PROCESSED FOODS

What is on your list that does not really fit into a Menu for Life shopping list category? Chances are good these items are packaged or processed, and convenience is their leading quality. Convenience is not always bad, of course, but read those labels! As a general rule, you want to stay away from processed foods and food kits. Foods to avoid include complete frozen dinners, canned goods, meals and side dishes that come in boxes with flavoring packets, or "instant" meals to which you simply add ground beef or a can of tuna. Instant lunch products, those noodle or rice "soups" to which you just add hot water, often contain half a day's sodium. Products such as these may appear to save you time, but the small amount of convenience they deliver is offset by the large amount of sodium these products contain. If you are using this type of processed food, you have to judge whether the high calories, sodium, fat, and lower overall nutrient content are worth adding to your Menu for Life Meal Planner for that day's eating. Remember your daily sodium target is 2,000 milligrams per day.

Some frozen pizzas and pizza kits can have as many as 350 calories *per serving*! That's 700 calories for only two slices of pizza, 1,050 calories for three slices! That is a lot when your daily calorie target is 1,800 to 2,400 calories a day. Frozen pizza and pizza kits tend to be high in sodium and sugar too. If you want pizza, you can have pizza. But read labels and make nutritious choices. Better yet, make your own. A prepared pizza crust (often found in the bakery department or in the frozen food section) is one ready-made product that can be worth buying. It is convenient, speeds cooking at home, and is available without a lot of sodium and fat. Instead of buying a pizza "kit" with its high-fat components, get a pizza crust, some fresh veggies, and make the Cold Vegetable Pizza recipe in this book.

If you haven't guessed by now, prepared food products you buy in a food kit, spoon from a can, or pop ready-made into the oven, such as complete frozen dinners, are actually things you can make easily and healthfully at home for yourself. For instance, pasta with a nice Italian tomato sauce. Cook your pasta ahead of time. Make a simple, nutrient-dense red sauce with fresh tomatoes. Add your own herbs and spice it up the way you like it. Divide the pasta and the sauce into individual servings, slip each serving into a little freezer bag or freezable container, and stack them in your freezer. When you need a quick meal, all you have to do is heat up one portion. This is a healthier way for you to eat. It's also better for your children. For a different kind of pasta sauce, try the recipe for Spaghetti with Pesto Sauce. Making your own is much better and more healthful than relying on bottled pasta sauces. Canned pasta products? Leave them on the shelf. Frozen Italian dinners (or *any* kind of frozen dinner)? Pass them by.

The same is true for canned soups. One serving of canned soup or chili can have as much as 1,050 milligrams of sodium, and that's a lot. Even the brands that are marketed as "healthy" can contain more sodium than you want to eat in one meal. Be aware that many cans of soup are considered two or more servings. When you read the label to check the fat, sodium, and total calories, you should also note how many servings are in each can. Four hundred and eighty milligrams of sodium may not sound so bad, but if the can contains two servings and you eat the whole can yourself, you've just had 960 milligrams of sodium in your soup alone. You can whip up a quick and easy soup yourself. When you have some time, you can make some Savory Vegetable Stock. (Yes, we've got a recipe for that too.) Add a package of frozen mixed vegetables, some seasoning, and you have a nice nutritious soup. Remember, the frozen vegetables will have a higher nutrient density than the canned soup's vegetables. If you want, you can freeze individual portions of your soup to eat later. Any time you need a quick meal, all you have to do is open the freezer, grab a soup container, and pop it in the microwave. Try the Gold Nugget Carrot Soup, made using fresh vegetables; it is easy and you will love it.

Now we arrive at the soda and snack foods, chips and such. If you must have them, you can work these items into your meal planner as special treats for special occasions—not every day (or even every week!) items. Pick baked chips over fried ones, low or no sodium over those with generous portions of sodium. Avoid chips made with fat substitutes. These "fake" fat products may have fewer calories, but they can wreak havoc with your digestive system and leave you feeling unsatisfied to boot! If you are going to buy chips, buy a small bag. Put a few chips on your plate with your sandwich, close the bag, and put the bag back on the shelf *before* you sit down to eat.

The sugar in soda translates into empty and unsatisfying calories, and diet soda has no calories but still contains sodium. Why not eat a piece of nutrient-dense fresh fruit instead and drink a tall glass of mineral water or iced tea you've brewed yourself with no added refined sugar? This satisfies your urge for something sweet and wet. For even better nutrient density and a super satisfying taste why not buy a variety of fruits and make a fruit salad? Of course, fruit juices are another option, but, as is the case with all processed foods, read the label carefully. When you look for juice, make sure the juice you are buying does not contain added sugar. Avoid "juice drinks." Juice drinks contain mostly water and sugar or high fructose corn syrup, another form of sugar and a source of empty unsatisfying calories. Sugar water fails the Menu for Life definition of juice! Make sure your juices are 100 percent fruit juices. Better yet, make fruit smoothies in your blender with some fresh fruit; add ice for coldness, yogurt for thickness, or soy milk for silkiness.

FAMILY SHOPPING

When you follow the Menu for Life guidelines, you no longer have to buy and make special foods for family members concerned about health problems such as diabetes, hypertension, or high cholesterol. One way of eating—the Menu for Life way—works for all. Having one plan that works for the whole family makes your shopping and cooking easier and helps you save money too. Who does the grocery shopping in your family? Often it is the same person who does the cooking . . . who is the same person who does the meal planning. Whether this is you or someone else in your family, *stick with your shopping list.* Your list protects you . . . even from your own family members who might plead for this or beg for that. If you can tell them consistently, "It's not on the list," before long they will work with you to get what they want to eat onto the list (anything is possible with your Menu for Life, as long as you work it sensibly into your

Meal Planner), or they will know that their in-store appeals will fail to sway you.

Shopping with children can be educational for the child and frustrating for you. You can help your child learn by example, as he or she watches you follow your list, read labels, and make nutritionally sound decisions. Some kids do well with this and enjoy participating. Others obsess about whatever they last saw on television, heard on the radio, had at a friend's house . . . and have to have *now*. Children have very poor impulse control. When shopping with a child, you may find he or she grabs a big bag of cookies or a box of sugary cereal and adds it to your cart. It can be tempting to allow one of those poor food choices to remain in your cart, just to keep your child happy and quiet. We can't tell you not to do this, but we *can* tell you that every time you do it you reinforce your child's expectation that you will do it each and every time you go to the store. Many parents prefer to leave kids at home to avoid confrontations in the grocery store. If you choose to take your child shopping with you, it helps to plan your shopping trips for when you are relatively refreshed and relaxed. Avoid grocery shopping at the end of a long day, on your way home from errands or other activities with your child, or when you are both (or all) tired, hungry, and cranky!

When you buy special items as treats your children know are theirs alone, wait until you pay for the items before you allow your children to open the food or let them eat any of the food. Better yet, wait until you are home and seated at your kitchen table to eat the treat. This teaches your children first that something is yours only after you pay for it, and second that there is a proper time and place to eat and that time and place is not at the grocery store. As a reward for good behavior, forget the candy. Make good behavior a true adventure—let your child pick out an exotic fruit or vegetable. This is a great way to get kids to try out new foods and incorporate them into your whole family's Menu for Life as a shared and enjoyed, healthful mealtime experience.

PROCEED TO CHECKOUT: MENU FOR LIFE TRIUMPHS!

So you have everything on your Menu for Life shopping list and you are ready to check out. Are you home safe? Not quite! Most stores have lots of impulse buys—more temptations—placed near the register. Resist!

Know you have filled your shopping cart with a week's worth of healthful, nutritious food. You have lean meats, fresh fruits and vegetables, and a great variety of tastes and textures. You don't *need* all that junk food you have to look at while you wait in line to pay. Turn your back on it!

Once your groceries are bagged and you are on your way out the door, celebrate your Menu for Life shopping mission accomplished! You are on your way home to prepare delicious, flavorful, nutritious weekly meals that are healthful, filling, and satisfying for you and for your family. Smile and feel good. Your Menu for Life is taking shape beautifully. Cook, eat, and enjoy!

11

~~~~~~~~~

Cooking with Donna:
Recipes You Will Love

DONNA RANDALL ~~

"You *can* cook. Yes you can! Even if you don't believe it right now. I doubt if there were two people in the hundreds of people Dr. Randall and I have worked with who believed they could cook at the beginning of the Obesity Study. Everyone said, 'I *can't*.' 'I don't know how.' But the moment you realize that you *can* cook, that cooking healthful meals for yourself and your family is enjoyable and *easy* to do and doesn't take a lot of time, is the moment other challenges seem easier to manage as well. The first hurdle is getting over cooking. And believe me, once you start making these recipes, you won't want to go back to bland food from a box or a bag, or eat your meals out of a fast-food wrapper. Your creative thoughts and feelings about food will be working overtime for you, but this time to your *health benefit*, to experience all the new tastes and flavors of cooking and eating well when you follow your Menu for Life."

DR. RANDALL ~~

"The way you eat is important. *What* you eat, and *how much* is important. Eating a variety of healthful foods, of interesting meals, is *very* important. If someone tells you that to be healthy you can only drink a vanilla milkshake every day for the rest of your life—and that is all that you are going to get to nourish you—pretty quickly you are not going to like it, and, moreover, you are not going to *do* it. Variety is the spice of life. There are so many healthful foods and so many wonderful ways to put together surprising, satisfying meals for the whole family that look and taste good. But I don't need to say any more to convince you: Start cooking Donna's recipes and you will find out all on your own! There's no sacrifice here. The foods you will be eating are Donna's gift to you—a gift of food artistry. Now, you can be a food artist too. Enjoy!"

Baby Spinach Salad with Almonds, Mandarin Oranges, and Raspberry-Lemonade Vinaigrette

DONNA SAYS:

"When you make a salad with iceberg lettuce, that's not salad—that's water! Baby spinach is a sweet green and gives you a good, delicious iron source. A mature spinach leaf is more fibrous and needs to be cooked to soften and break it down, but not the baby spinach—and that makes it great for salads. You can buy a bunch and wash it yourself, but wash it well as it tends to contain some grit. Or, if it's worth it to you to save time and spend a little extra money, you can buy baby spinach pre-washed in bags. Then it's just a matter of grabbing a handful out of the bag and throwing it in the salad bowl!

"Adding fresh vegetables and other interesting, high-flavor additions like mandarin oranges and a sprinkle of almonds builds your salad, as we've done here. For the raspberries in the dressing, use fresh and just crush with a spoon or in a blender. To enjoy this recipe all year round, use frozen raspberries, but choose a brand that is frozen with no added sugar. Don't substitute raspberry jam in a pinch—the flavor and texture won't be right and the extra sugar spoils the dressing's tangy flavor.

"For different tastes, just vary the vegetables in your salad, or try a different dressing, like the Cinnamon Peach and Poppy Seed Vinaigrette or the Jalapeno Lime Vinaigrette dressings that follow. Just can't do without that taste of cheese? Try our version of Cheesy Pepper Dressing. These dressing flavors keep your salad interesting, flavorful, and nutrient dense—with no added fat, unnecessary or empty calories, or excess sugar. There's no reason a healthy salad has to be boring, and the more intense the flavor, the more you'll enjoy what you are eating."

SALAD

4 cups baby spinach
1 small bunch scallions (about 4), tops removed, thinly sliced
   about halfway up the green part
1 medium cucumber, peeled and thinly sliced
1 4-oz. can mandarin oranges, rinsed
1 tablespoon sliced almonds

DRESSING

1/2 cup lemonade
1 tablespoon cornstarch
1/2 cup raspberry vinegar or apple cider vinegar
1/2 cup crushed or pureed, fresh or frozen (without sugar)
   raspberries
1 tablespoon chopped fresh mint, or 1 teaspoon dried and crushed
   between your palms before adding
1 tablespoon minced scallions
Dash of black pepper

METHOD

1. To make the salad: wash and dry spinach, or remove from bag. Place in
   salad bowl and toss in the scallions, cucumber, mandarin oranges, and
   almonds.
2. To make the dressing: pour lemonade in a 1-quart saucepan and whisk
   in cornstarch with a wire whisk. Turn heat to medium and slowly whisk
   in vinegar. Heat, stirring constantly, until mixture thickens and begins
   to bubble, about 5 to 7 minutes.
3. Add the crushed or pureed raspberries. Bring mixture back to a boil, stir,
   and cook 1 minute longer.
4. Remove from heat. Stir in mint, scallions, and pepper. Cover and refrigerate for one hour or up to one week.

To serve the salad: Serve with the Raspberry-Lemonade Vinaigrette or any
of the dressings that follow. A serving of dressing is about 1 tablespoon,
and that may not seem like much, but if you serve it in a little dish on the
side and dip your fork in the dressing, then in the spinach, that dressing

(continued)

goes a long way. Or, measure 1/4 cup of dressing into the salad bowl and toss with the salad to make four ready-to-eat servings. Cover the remaining dressing in an airtight container to use throughout the week. This dressing should last in the refrigerator for about a week.

NUTRITIONAL INFORMATION PER SERVING
Calories 73
Total fat 1 g
Saturated fat .11 g
Unsaturated fat .81 g
Cholesterol 0
Sodium 35 mg
Carbohydrates 15 g
Protein 1.9 g
Food Exchange Value: 1 fruit, 1 vegetable

Honey Peach Vinaigrette

DONNA SAYS:
"The honey and cardamom do amazing things to the peach flavor in this dressing—and no worries about too much refined sugar or empty calories."

Serves about 16

1 tablespoon canola oil
2 tablespoons white wine vinegar
1/4 cup orange juice
1/4 cup peach or apricot nectar
1 tablespoon honey
1/4 teaspoon ground cardamom (or crush the seeds with a mortar
   and pestle)
1 large peach, peeled, pitted, and quartered

METHOD
1. Place all ingredients in a blender or food processor fitted with a steel blade. Blend or process on medium until smooth.

2. Cover and refrigerate at least 1 hour before serving. Cover and refrigerate any leftover dressing in an airtight container for up to one week.

NUTRITIONAL INFORMATION PER SERVING

Calories 20
Total Fat .9 g
Saturated Fat .06 g
Unsaturated Fat .79 g
Cholesterol 0
Sodium .40 mg
Carbohydrates 3.2 g
Protein .12 g
Food Exchange Value: free

Jalapeno Lime Vinaigrette

~~~~~~~~~~

DONNA SAYS:

"The one teaspoon of sugar in this dressing gives a hint of sweetness to balance the bite of the lime juice and jalapeno—and spread over eight servings, it doesn't amount to much."

Serves 8

1 tablespoon extra virgin olive oil
1 tablespoon balsamic vinegar
2 tablespoons freshly squeezed lime juice
1 tablespoon nonfat buttermilk
1 teaspoon sugar
2 tablespoons chopped fresh cilantro
1/2 small jalapeno, seeded, and very finely chopped

METHOD

1. Mix all ingredients until well blended. Serve 1 tablespoon over each serving of salad.
2. Cover and refrigerate any leftover dressing in an airtight container. It will keep for about three days, but it probably won't last that long!

(continued)

NUTRITIONAL INFORMATION PER SERVING

Calories 21

Total Fat 1.8 g

Saturated Fat .26 g

Unsaturated Fat 1.5 g

Cholesterol .08 mg

Sodium 2.9 mg

Carbohydrates 1.3 g

Protein .11 g

Food Exchange Value: free

Cheesy Pepper Dressing

DONNA SAYS:

"Here you get that creamy texture and cheese taste that satisfies, without the fat. The Parmesan adds a little bit of sodium, but not enough to get you into trouble, and the spices give this dressing a robust flavor."

Serves 16

1/2 cup plain nonfat yogurt

1/4 cup grated Parmesan

1/4 cup nonfat buttermilk

1 garlic clove, peeled and finely chopped

1 shallot, peeled and finely chopped, or 2 tablespoons minced yellow onion

1 teaspoon oregano

1/4 teaspoon black pepper

METHOD

1. Put all ingredients in a blender or a glass jar with a screw-top lid.
2. Blend or shake until well combined, about 30 seconds.
3. Cover and refrigerate any leftover dressing in an airtight container. It should keep for about a week.

NUTRITIONAL INFORMATION PER SERVING

Calories 11.7
Total Fat .43 g
Saturated Fat .27 g
Unsaturated Fat .13 g
Cholesterol 1.4 mg
Sodium 31.7 mg
Carbohydrates 1.1 g
Protein 1 g
Food Exchange Value: free

Sweet-Tart Fruit Salad

DONNA SAYS:

"This special fruit salad uses sweet fruits and tart balsamic vinegar. Yes, vinegar! Strange as it may sound, balsamic vinegar has an amazing effect on fresh fruit, drawing out the maximum fruity flavor. Serve this on a bed of nutritious and crunchy salad greens for a light lunch or a surprisingly elegant first course. Serve in pretty glass bowls for an impressive dessert. Use all fresh fruits for the best texture, but don't be afraid to substitute different fruits if the ones in this recipe are out of season."

Serves 6

1 cup fresh strawberries, hulled and cut in half
1 cup blackberries or black raspberries
1 cup cantaloupe chunks (about 1-inch cubes or balls)
1 cup honeydew chunks (about 1-inch cubes or balls)
2 seedless oranges cut in half, then sliced (you can substitute 1 can
    mandarin oranges, drained)
1/4 cup balsamic vinegar
6 cups salad greens (like romaine, Boston, or bibb lettuce or baby
    spinach, not iceberg lettuce), washed and dried

(continued)

METHOD

1. Toss the strawberries, blackberries or black raspberries, cantaloupe, honeydew, and oranges together in a large bowl.
2. Sprinkle with balsamic vinegar and toss gently.
3. Serve on a bed of salad greens, on individual plates, or on a big platter.

NUTRITIONAL INFORMATION PER SERVING

Calories 7 g
Total Fat .5 g
Saturated Fat .06 g
Unsaturated Fat .26 g
Cholesterol 0
Sodium 24.3 mg
Carbohydrates 19 g
Protein 1.8 g
Food Exchange Value: 1 fruit, 1 vegetable

Herb Garden Dip

DONNA SAYS:

"Use Herb Garden Dip with raw vegetables: carrots, broccoli, cauliflower, whatever you like. You'll love the creamy taste and the colorful appearance. It's a great way to inspire you to eat more vegetables. You can also use this more substantial dressing as a sauce over cold chicken or fish for your dinner meal, but in that case, stick to about a tablespoon per serving instead of the 1/4 cup serving used for dipping."

Makes 2 cups (about 8 servings as dip or 32 servings as sauce)

1 cup plain nonfat yogurt
1/2 cup nonfat ricotta cheese
1/4 cup nonfat mayonnaise
1 teaspoon Dijon or other brown mustard
1/4 cup green onions with tops, chopped

1/4 cup minced red bell pepper

1/4 cup finely chopped fresh baby spinach or other leafy green

1 tablespoon capers or chopped green or black olives (whichever
   you like best)

1 tablespoon fresh parsley, chopped (or 1 teaspoon dried)

1 tablespoon fresh dill, chopped (or 1 teaspoon dried)

1 tablespoon fresh tarragon, chopped (or 1 teaspoon dried)

2 garlic cloves, crushed

1/2 teaspoon paprika

Dash of freshly ground pepper

2 tablespoons nonfat buttermilk or skim milk (if texture is too stiff)

METHOD

1. Put yogurt, ricotta cheese, and mayonnaise in a mixing bowl or food
   processor and mix or process until well blended, about 30 seconds.
2. Add remaining ingredients except milk. Stir with a fork until combined.
   Add buttermilk or milk if the dip is too stiff.
3. Cover and chill for one hour or up to 24 hours before serving.
4. Refrigerate leftover dip for up to three days.

NUTRITIONAL INFORMATION PER SERVING

Calories 48

Total Fat 1.5 g

Saturated Fat .84 g

Unsaturated Fat .43 g

Cholesterol 0

Sodium 137 mg

Carbohydrates 5.8 g

Protein 3.9 g

Food Exchange Value: 1/2 milk

Spaghetti with Pesto Sauce

~~~~~~~~

DONNA SAYS:

"A cup of pasta with a highly flavored sauce is a delicious and filling meal. It's easy to think you need more than a cup of pasta because so many restaurants serve you three and four times that much, but once you eat a cup with a good sauce and stop, you will recognize that you're actually satisfied, especially with this pesto sauce that looks fancy but is really easy to make and has no oil."

Makes 8 servings

16-oz. package spaghetti
1 10-oz. bag baby spinach or about 8 cups of spinach, washed with
    stems removed
1 cup nonfat cottage cheese
4 garlic cloves, minced
1 tablespoon dried basil
1 tablespoon Parmesan cheese
Dash of black pepper
1/2 cup nonfat buttermilk, or enough to make a smooth texture

METHOD
1. Cook spaghetti according to package directions until tender but firm (called "al dente"). Drain in a colander and set aside.
2. Place all remaining ingredients except the buttermilk in a food processor and blend for one full minute. Scrape down the sides of the food processing container with a rubber scraper.
3. Add about half the buttermilk and process an additional one minute. If the sauce is still too thick to toss with pasta, add the remaining buttermilk and process just to combine, about 15–30 seconds.
4. Place spaghetti in a large bowl. Top with pesto sauce and toss until spaghetti noodles are coated with sauce.

OPTIONS
• Serve this hot for dinner or cold for a nice summer lunch. It's delicious both ways.

• Substitute different kinds of pasta for the spaghetti. Macaroni or other stubby pasta mixed with pesto sauce and chilled makes a nice pasta salad, especially if you add some chopped raw vegetables like grated carrots, diced tomatoes, and broccoli florets.

NUTRITIONAL INFORMATION PER SERVING

Calories 251
Total Fat 1.4 g
Saturated Fat .36 g
Unsaturated Fat .63 g
Cholesterol 2.7 mg
Sodium 185 mg
Carbohydrates 46.6 g
Protein 12.5 g
Food Exchange Value: 3 starch/bread, 2 milk

Savory Vegetable Stock

DONNA SAYS:

"Vegetable stock makes a great base for soups and enriches any savory recipe as a replacement for water (see the Gold Nugget Carrot Soup recipe as a perfect example of where to use this stock). To simplify this recipe when you have less time, substitute a 16-ounce bag of frozen mixed vegetables along with an onion and a couple of cloves of garlic to make this stock.

"Instead of straining the stock, you can also leave the vegetables in and puree in batches after cooking to make a nice vegetable sauce that tastes great over meatloaf. Freeze in 1-cup portions to serve 4, or in ice cube trays for individual servings. If you don't freeze it, you can keep stock for up to one week in the refrigerator."

Yields one gallon

2 medium yellow potatoes, eyes removed, unpeeled, cut into 2-inch cubes
2 medium yellow or white onions, peeled and thickly sliced
4 cloves of garlic, peeled and minced or thinly sliced

(continued)

4 celery stalks, sliced, including tops

1 cup sliced mushrooms (portabello and shitake have the highest nutritional value, but if you can't find them, use the common white button mushrooms)

8 carrots, scrubbed and thickly sliced

4 stalks celery, coarsely chopped

1/2 cup chopped fresh parsley or cilantro (remove stems)

2 bay leaves

2 tablespoons fresh basil, chopped, or 2 teaspoons dried and crushed

1 tablespoon fresh oregano, chopped, or 1 teaspoon dried and crushed

Dash cayenne pepper or 1/4 teaspoon red pepper flakes (optional, but good if you like your stock spicy)

METHOD

1. Place all ingredients in a 2-gallon capacity stock pot and cover with one gallon of water. Bring to a boil over high heat, then reduce heat to medium and simmer uncovered for 45 minutes to 1 hour.
2. Turn off heat and allow mixture to steep an additional 15–30 minutes.
3. Carefully pour the stock through a colander into a large bowl. Discard vegetables (or save them and puree with stock as described in the directions above, but wait until they are cooled to puree them).
4. Store stock in quart size containers. Leave an inch or two of space at the top if you want to freeze the stock for future use, or store in the refrigerator for up to one week.

NUTRITIONAL INFORMATION PER SERVING

Calories 43

Total Fat .17 g

Saturated Fat .03 g

Unsaturated Fat .09 g

Cholesterol 0

Sodium 36 mg

Carbohydrates 9.8 g

Protein 1.3 g

Food Exchange Value: 1/2 vegetable

Gold Nugget Carrot Soup

DONNA SAYS:

"This soup is light and elegant, perfect for company or a light but special lunch. It has a unique flavor that is surprisingly sweet and rich, considering it has virtually no fat."

Serves 6

1 medium yellow onion, peeled and chopped
2 cloves garlic, peeled and minced
4 carrots, scrubbed and thickly sliced
1 tablespoon grated fresh ginger or 1 teaspoon dried powdered
    ginger
1 tablespoon cumin
1/2 teaspoon cinnamon
1/4 teaspoon nutmeg
6 cups low sodium vegetable stock or low sodium, fat-free chicken
    broth
1/4 cup nonfat buttermilk

GARNISH

2 carrots, scrubbed and chopped into small dice (the "nuggets")
    (about 1 cup)
nonfat sour cream
dried cumin

METHOD

1. Spray a soup pot or Dutch oven with nonstick cooking spray and add onions, garlic, and carrots. Heat over medium heat until onions are soft and carrots are fork-tender, about 10 minutes.
2. Add ginger, cumin, cinnamon, and nutmeg, and stir into onion/carrot mixture for one minute.
3. Add vegetable or chicken stock and stir to combine. Increase heat to medium-high and heat until soup boils. Reduce heat to low, cover, and simmer for 30 minutes.

(continued)

4. Remove from heat and allow soup to cool for about 30 to 45 minutes. When lukewarm, puree in blender or food processor.
5. Return to soup or stock pot and heat over medium heat until heated through, about ten minutes.
6. Stir in buttermilk, reduce heat to low, and heat for an additional 5 minutes.
7. Ladle into soup bowls. Top each bowl with a teaspoon of nonfat sour cream, a sprinkle of cubed raw carrots, and a dash of cumin.

NUTRITIONAL INFORMATION PER SERVING

Calories 44
Total Fat 1.1 g
Saturated Fat .19 g
Unsaturated Fat .56 g
Cholesterol .63 mg
Sodium 141 mg
Carbohydrates 7.6 g
Protein 1.6 g
Food Exchange Value: 1/2 vegetable

Vegetarian Chili

DONNA SAYS:
"Chili is a great one-pot meal that provides so much variety and nutrient density. Make a pot and the whole family can enjoy it all week."

Serves 12

1 cup dried kidney beans (or substitute a 15- or 16-oz. can, drained and rinsed)
1 cup dried pinto beans (or substitute a 15- or 16-oz. can, drained and rinsed)
1 cup dried navy beans (or substitute a 15- or 16-oz. can navy or other white beans, drained and rinsed)
1 white onion, chopped

4 cloves garlic, finely chopped

2 red bell peppers, seeded and chopped

2 green bell peppers, seeded and chopped

1/2 small jalapeno, seeded and finely chopped (optional, but good
   if you like your chili spicy)

2 tablespoons chili powder

1 tablespoon ground cumin

1 tablespoon finely chopped fresh basil, or 2 teaspoons dried

1 32-oz. can tomatoes, chopped, plus their juices

1 cup red wine or dark beer

4 cups low sodium vegetable stock

GARNISH

nonfat sour cream

fresh chopped cilantro

diced fresh tomato

METHOD

1. Put all the dried beans in a bowl and cover them with about three inches of water. Soak for 12 hours or overnight.

2. Drain, discard soaking water, and put the beans in a 4-qt. soup pot or Dutch oven and cover with fresh water.

3. Cook over medium heat until the water boils. Reduce heat and simmer until beans are tender, about 2 hours.

4. Put onions, garlic, bell peppers, and jalapeno in a Dutch oven sprayed with nonstick cooking spray and sauté on medium-high heat for about 5 minutes or until just beginning to soften.

5. Add chili powder, cumin, basil, canned tomatoes and juice, wine, or beer, cooked beans if you started with dried beans (don't add canned beans yet), and vegetable stock to the vegetables and continue to cook over medium-high heat until boiling. Reduce heat and simmer for 30 minutes.

6. If you are using canned beans, add them now and simmer an additional 10 minutes to heat through.

7. Ladle into bowls and garnish with a dollop of sour cream sprinkled with fresh cilantro and diced tomatoes.

(continued)

NUTRITIONAL INFORMATION PER SERVING

Calories 232

Total Fat 1.6 g

Saturated Fat .44 g

Unsaturated Fat .55 g

Cholesterol 1.28 mg

Sodium 186 mg

Carbohydrates 40 g

Protein 14 g

Food Exchange Value: 2 1/2 vegetable, 2 very lean meat

Roasted Niçoise Salad

DONNA SAYS:

"Traditionally, Niçoise salad uses tuna, although some variations use salmon or chicken. This one is a perfect side dish because it doesn't include any meat, poultry, or fish, making it very low in fat, but high in fiber and nutrition. It's also an excellent way to use the bountiful produce at farmer's markets and roadside produce stands in the summer.

"This recipe has a large yield, perfect for entertaining or for extended family dinners. If you are cooking for only yourself or a small group, you can freeze leftovers in individual portions as a perfect side to a quick-grilled piece of chicken for an easy dinner after a long day. Or serve leftovers over rice for a light dinner. Or to serve only four, cut the recipe in half."

Serves 8

SALAD

1 lb fresh green beans, ends trimmed off

1 lb new potatoes, scrubbed but unpeeled (cut out any bad spots or
   eyes) and quartered

1 red bell pepper, cored, seeded, and sliced into strips

1 yellow bell pepper, cored, seeded, and sliced into strips

1 teaspoon Italian seasoning or 1/2 teaspoon basil and 1/2 teaspoon oregano

3 fresh, ripe tomatoes, cored and diced

8 green olives, sliced

3 hardboiled eggs, cut in half, yolks removed, then coarsely chopped

5 green onions, tops removed, chopped including part of the greens

DRESSING

1 tablespoon olive oil

2 tablespoons freshly squeezed lemon juice

1 teaspoon Dijon or other brown mustard

1 tablespoon chopped fresh parsley

Black pepper

METHOD

1. Preheat oven to 400° F.
2. Spray a roasting pan with nonstick cooking spray. Spread green beans, potatoes, and peppers in the pan. Spray the vegetables again lightly with nonstick cooking spray and sprinkle with Italian seasoning or basil and oregano.
3. Bake for 45 minutes or until potatoes are nicely browned and fork-tender.
4. Put roasted vegetables into a large bowl. Add the tomatoes, olives, eggs, and green onion. Toss to combine.
5. In a small bowl or glass jar with a screw-top lid, combine olive oil, lemon juice, mustard, parsley, and black pepper. Whisk with a wire whisk or shake until well combined. Pour over vegetables. Toss to coat.
6. Serve warm or chill for 2 hours and serve cold. It's delicious both ways. Or have it warm one night and cold the next day for lunch!

OPTIONS

To make this more like a traditional Niçoise salad and a main dish meal, add 1 drained can of reduced-sodium tuna, salmon, or chicken to the bowl just before adding the dressing. Toss to combine.

(continued)

NUTRITIONAL INFORMATION PER SERVING
   Calories 92
   Total fat 2.6 g
   Saturated fat .34 g
   Unsaturated fat 1.9 g
   Cholesterol 0
   Sodium 128 mg
   Carbohydrates 15 g
   Protein 3.6 g
   Food Exchange Value: 1 starchy vegetable, 1/2 medium fat meat, 1/2 fat

Cold Fresh Vegetable Pizza

DONNA SAYS:

"Cold fresh vegetable pizza is very easy to make. Use a prepared pizza crust from the grocery store. Overall, you can reduce the fat and sodium content of the prepared crust by increasing the number of slices for smaller individual servings. We've done this pizza countless times in cooking demonstrations and everyone loves it. Spread, layer, slice, and you've got a beautiful cold pizza in the summer to serve—cold and fresh."

Serves 4–6 as lunch or 12 as an appetizer

1 prepared pizza crust (such as Boboli)
1/2 cup nonfat yogurt
1/2 cup nonfat sour cream
1 garlic clove, minced
1 tablespoon fresh dill
1 tablespoon fresh basil, chopped
1/4 teaspoon red pepper flakes (optional, but good if you like it a little spicy)
1 bell pepper (any color, or a combination of colors), sliced in thin rings
1 cup broccoli florets sliced into bite-sized pieces
1/2 cup baby carrots sliced into matchsticks or disks

1/2 cup chopped fresh tomatoes

1/2–1 cup of any other vegetables you like raw, such as cauliflower, mushrooms, chopped fresh spinach, or raw peas fresh from the garden

1 tablespoon chopped green or black olives or capers (optional, adds 79 mg sodium per serving)

1/4 cup marinated artichoke hearts, drained and chopped (optional, adds 121 mg sodium per serving)

1/2 cup low-sodium, lowfat mozzarella cheese

1/4 teaspoon paprika

METHOD

1. Place the pizza crust on a plate or cutting board. In a small bowl, mix yogurt, sour cream, garlic, fresh dill, fresh basil, and optional red pepper flakes together. Spread onto pizza crust.

2. Top pizza with pepper rings. Then arrange broccoli, carrots, tomatoes, any other vegetables you like, and optional olives or capers or artichoke hearts over the pepper rings. Sprinkle with mozzarella cheese and paprika. Cut with a sharp knife or pizza cutter into 12 slices.

NUTRITIONAL INFORMATION PER SERVING

	Lunch	*Appetizer*
Calories	303	101
Total fat	5.4 g	1.81 g
Saturated fat	1.6 g	.54 g
Unsaturated fat	1.1 g	.37 g
Cholesterol	8.3 mg	2.8 mg
Sodium	628 mg	209 mg
Carbohydrates	48 g	16.1 g
Protein	14.5 g	4.8 g

Food Exchange Value:

Lunch: 2 starch/bread, 1 vegetable, 1 milk, 1 medium-fat meat, 1 fat

Appetizer: 2/3 starch/bread, 1/3 vegetable, 1/3 milk, 1/3 medium-fat meat, 1/3 fat

Broiled Citrus Swordfish with Caribbean Chutney

~~~~~~~~~

DONNA SAYS:

"Swordfish works for me in this recipe because it doesn't have that strong, fishy taste, but it has a great flavor. Because swordfish flesh is firm and easy to work with you can butterfly, grill, broil, or bake it without being concerned that it will break, or fall apart when you turn it. Any meaty fish will also work with this recipe, such as grouper or salmon.

"The citrus juices used on the fish in this recipe will always taste best if freshly squeezed, but if you don't have fresh limes on hand or if grapefruits are out of season, bottled will still work.

"This Caribbean chutney is nice, its exotic fruits make it both tart and sweet. These days you can find all these tropical fruits in the grocery store without a problem. This chutney has other uses, as well—try it over other meats like a lean pork loin, or as a snack on wheat crackers with a little nonfat cream cheese."

Serves 6

BROILED CITRUS SWORDFISH

6 swordfish steaks, 1-inch thick, about 4 ounces each
1/4 cup lime juice
1/4 cup pineapple juice
1/4 cup ruby red grapefruit juice
1 tablespoon rum (optional) or 1 tablespoon sodium-reduced soy
    sauce
2 tablespoons grated lime peel
1 tablespoon grated ginger (for best taste, grate a ginger root, but
    dried will also work in a pinch)
1 garlic clove, crushed
1/4 teaspoon allspice

CARIBBEAN CHUTNEY

1/4 cup finely chopped fresh tomato
1 tablespoon finely chopped yellow or red bell pepper (or green if
    you can't find the others)
1 papaya, peeled, seeded, and chopped

1 mango, peeled, seeded, and chopped

1/4 cup lime juice

1 tablespoon lemon juice

1/4 cup finely chopped green onions

1 tablespoon chopped fresh cilantro (or 1 teaspoon dried, but fresh
is easy to find and tastes much better)

METHOD

1. First, marinate your fish for maximum flavor. Put the swordfish (or whatever fish you are using) in an ungreased ceramic casserole or glass baking dish, about 8 inches in diameter. Combine the juices, rum, or soy sauce, lime peel, ginger, garlic, and allspice in a small bowl. Remove and reserve 1/4 cup of the marinade in a covered container and store it in the refrigerator for when you are cooking the fish. Cover the casserole or baking dish and refrigerate the fish for 2 hours or up to 12 hours.

2. Now make the chutney. Combine all the ingredients in a medium bowl, mixing gently but thoroughly (to avoid smashing up or bruising the fruit too much). Cover and refrigerate for at least one hour, so the flavors can blend, but make sure to serve it within one day.

3. Now it's time to cook the fish. Place the oven rack about 6 inches from the broiler coils and preheat the broiler. Spray the broiler pan with non-stick cooking spray. Remove the fish from the marinade and discard the marinade. Broil fish for about 8 minutes, turn, and broil another 4 minutes.

4. Pull broiler pan out of the oven and brush the remaining reserved marinade over the top of the fish. Return fish to broiler and broil an additional 5 minutes, or until fish flakes easily with a fork.

GARNISH

Remove fish to a platter or individual plates and top each fish steak with about 1/3 cup of chutney.

OPTIONS

• Experiment with different kinds of fish in this recipe: halibut, salmon, or tuna steaks. It's also good with pork loin or chicken breast.

• Can't find one of the tropical fruits? Double the mango or the papaya or substitute pineapple, kiwi, or even bananas.

(continued)

NUTRITIONAL INFORMATION PER SERVING

Calories 241

Total fat 6.2 g

Saturated fat 1.7 g

Unsaturated fat 3.8 g

Cholesterol 57 mg

Sodium 253 mg

Carbohydrates 16.5 g

Protein 30 g

Food Exchange Value: 1 fruit, 4 lean meat, 1 fat

Spicy Scallop Roll

DONNA SAYS:

"This is a light dish that sounds like the sushi dish by the same name, but don't be fooled. No raw fish here, this is all cooked and delicious, and wrapped in crunchy lettuce leaves. I serve it with a brown rice or a rice pilaf containing both white and wild rice. If you use a store-bought red pepper sauce, check the label for low sodium content and the least amount of preservatives; or, you can use just a pinch (about 1/4 teaspoon) of crushed red pepper flakes, if that is easier or more convenient. The taste of fresh cilantro is one you will savor; it's worth the trouble to get this herb fresh— and these days, it's not much trouble since you can usually find it in any grocery store. Look next to the fresh parsley. If your grocery store doesn't carry it, try your local health food store or specialty market. If you absolutely can't find fresh cilantro, you can substitute fresh parsley or fresh Italian parsley, although it won't be quite the same. Don't bother with dried cilantro and don't jump to substitute for fresh cilantro—put on your walking shoes and be persistent; you'll be glad you did."

2 red bell peppers, seeded and quartered

2 cloves garlic, peeled

1/4 cup packed fresh cilantro leaves, stems removed

1 tablespoon freshly squeezed lemon juice

1/4 teaspoon hot pepper sauce

1 pound cooked scallops (or buy them raw and sauté with nonstick cooking spray over medium-high heat until white in the center, about 5 minutes)

1/4 cup thinly sliced scallion or white onion

1/4 cup finely chopped celery

12 large leaves of soft lettuce like Boston or butter lettuce

12 toothpicks

METHOD

1. Put the red peppers and garlic in a large microwavable bowl or casserole. Cover with plastic wrap or casserole lid and microwave on high for 10 minutes. No need to add any water.

2. Remove from microwave and put peppers and garlic in a blender or food processor fitted with the steel blade. Add cilantro, lemon juice, and hot pepper sauce. Process until well combined, about 1 minute.

3. In a large bowl, put cooked scallops, scallions or onion, and celery. Toss to combine. Add the red bell pepper–garlic mixture and toss to coat.

4. Working with one roll at a time, put a lettuce leaf on a plate. Put 1/12th of the scallop/sauce mixture on the leaf, roll up, and secure with a toothpick. Continue until you have 12 rolls.

5. Serve each person 3 rolls for a delicious main course.

NUTRITIONAL INFORMATION PER SERVING

Calories 152

Total fat 3.9 g

Saturated fat .66 g

Unsaturated fat 2.6 g

Cholesterol 36.6 mg

Sodium 23.3 mg

Carbohydrates 9.3 g

Protein 20 g

Food Exchange Value: 1/2 vegetable, 3 very lean meat, 1/2 fat

Oven-Fried Cajun Catfish

~~~~~~~~

DONNA SAYS:

"We know you love your fried fish. Well, here it is. You don't have to cheat to get it. We promise you, it will satisfy."

DR. RANDALL SAYS:

"I like the taste of this recipe. Whether it is fish or chicken, once you get the skin off the seasoning gets right into the meat. Oven-fried with cornmeal is better, healthier. You don't lose anything in the taste, you gain something. It's cleaner. The consistency of the cornmeal that is put into this batter makes it almost like a skin."

DONNA SAYS:

"Don't fall into the trap that more cornmeal gives you a *more fried* taste. Follow the recipe and you will get the fried texture you are looking for. Make sure all the meat is covered, but you don't want to see dry, caked spots of extra cornmeal. On fish, the thinnest possible coating works best."

DR. RANDALL SAYS:

"It's still crispy and still good—the consistency of the coating makes it nice."

DONNA SAYS:

"Use a prepared salt-free Cajun seasoning (Cajun blends with salt have too high a sodium content), or experiment and create your own blend, spicy or mild, or use the homemade recipe after this recipe. Oven frying with cornmeal and cooking spray offers everything deep frying or pan frying does with the exception of added fat. Our method provides you with fish that is crispy on the outside and moist on the inside. Serve your oven-fried catfish with potatoes, rice, vegetables—whatever you like. You choose."

Serves 4

1/4 cup skim milk
2 tablespoons *salt-free* Cajun seasoning, divided in half (try the recipe below)
1/2 cup yellow cornmeal
4 catfish fillets, 4 oz. each

METHOD

1. Preheat the oven to 350° F. Spray a baking sheet with the non-stick cooking spray. Try the kind flavored like garlic for an extra kick.
2. Put the milk in a shallow dish and sprinkle with one tablespoon of the Cajun seasoning. Whisk with a fork.
3. Put the cornmeal in a shallow dish or pie plate and combine with the other tablespoon of Cajun seasoning. Mix with a fork until well combined and sprinkle half the mixture evenly over the baking sheet.
4. Take each catfish fillet, dip into the spicy milk mix on both sides, then place the fillets on the baking sheet so they aren't touching each other.
5. Sprinkle the remaining cornmeal mixture lightly and evenly over the top of each fillet to get that thin coating.
6. Spray the tops of the fish with non-stick cooking spray and bake for about 40 minutes, or until the topping is lightly browned and looks crispy.

HOMEMADE *SALT-FREE* CAJUN SEASONING

This recipe makes just over one cup. Keep it in a jar and store with your other spices or store it in an empty salt shaker to add a zesty Cajun flavor to any meat you are cooking.

4 tablespoons black pepper
4 tablespoons cayenne pepper
4 tablespoons chili powder
2 tablespoons garlic powder
1 tablespoon onion powder
1 tablespoon dried parsley flakes, crushed
1 teaspoon nutmeg
1 teaspoon dried thyme

Thoroughly combine all spices/herbs and store in a glass jar.

NUTRITIONAL INFORMATION PER SERVING

Calories 260
Total fat 11.25 g
Saturated fat 2.6 g
Unsaturated fat 7.5 g
Cholesterol 68 mg

(continued)

Sodium 76 mg
Carbohydrates 15.9 g
Protein 25.2 g
Food Exchange Value: 1 starch/bread, 4 lean meat, 1/2 milk, 1/2 fat

Potato Sausage Pie

DONNA SAYS:

"There are a lot of ways to go about getting the turkey sausage for this recipe. If you are using store-bought sausage, look for the brand with the lowest fat and sodium content on the label. If you can buy your sausage at a farmer's market, you may find sausages made with organic meat and hand-prepared seasonings. (How about planning a summer day-trip with the kids? Who knows what other good foods you'll find at the market! That's a fun day of walking and discovering new, fresh ingredients for your family's meals.) Or, you can make your own sausage equivalent at home by buying a pound of ground turkey (ask the butcher to grind a turkey breast because the regular ground kind can have a lot of fat) and mix in your own, individualized blend of your favorite Italian seasonings, to taste, such as oregano, basil, garlic powder, even a little cayenne pepper for a kick. When you make it at home, *you* control the additives that go into your meat; you don't have to let someone do this for you—you have a choice. Serve your meal with steamed vegetables."

Serves 8

6 medium-sized red potatoes, scrubbed, peeled, eyes removed
1/2 pound Italian turkey sausage, or 1 pound ground turkey plus
    2 tablespoons Italian seasonings
2 tablespoons reduced-sodium grated Parmesan cheese
1 large yellow onion, peeled and thinly sliced
1/2 cup nonfat buttermilk
1 tablespoon mustard
1/4 teaspoon garlic powder (not garlic salt)
Dash of black pepper
1/4 cup toasted dry bread crumbs
1/8 teaspoon nutmeg

METHOD

1. Preheat oven to 350° F.
2. Cut potatoes in half immediately after peeling, and put them directly into a soup pot or Dutch oven with about 8 cups of water, to keep them from discoloring. Turn heat to medium-high and bring water to a boil. Boil potatoes until fork-tender, about 30 minutes depending on the size of the potato chunks.
3. While the potatoes are boiling, remove sausage from casing or, if preparing your own meat, mix ground turkey with Italian seasonings, by hand or in a food processor. Cook sausage in a medium saucepan over medium heat until well browned, about 20 minutes.
4. Drain potatoes and carefully move them to a cutting board. When they are cool enough to handle, slice them as thin as you can.
5. Spray a 9-inch deep dish pie plate or 2-qt. casserole with nonstick cooking spray. Using 1/3 of the potato slices, arrange a layer of potato on the bottom of the plate. Sprinkle with half the cheese. Cover with a layer made from half the sliced onions, followed by a layer of half the sausage. Repeat using another layer of potatoes, cheese, onions, sausage, then the final layer of potatoes.
6. Heat the milk in a 1-cup glass measuring cup in the microwave for 1 minute. Whisk in the mustard, garlic powder, and black pepper, then pour this mixture over the pie.
7. Toss breadcrumbs with nutmeg in a small bowl, then sprinkle over the top of the casserole.
8. Bake for 1 hour. To serve, cut into wedges or squares.

NUTRITIONAL INFORMATION PER SERVING

Calories 125
Total fat 4 g
Saturated fat 1.4 g
Unsaturated fat 2.5 g
Cholesterol 25 mg
Sodium 330 mg
Carbohydrates 15.5 g
Protein 7.5 g
Food Exchange Value: 1 starchy vegetable, 1 medium-fat meat

PORK LOIN 3 WAYS:
Baked Stuffed Pork Loin;
Barbecue Pulled Pork Sandwiches;
Vegetable Pork Stir-Fry Medley

DONNA SAYS:

"People come to me and say, 'Donna, I want my pork chops.' I say *never* buy pork chops, buy the center cut, the pork loin. Why buy all that bone and all that fat? You're just paying for it to go in the garbage. Look at what your money buys with a pork chop and what it buys with pork loin. You can eat *all* of the pork loin, every dime of it."

Each recipe serves 4

Baked Stuffed Pork Loin

DONNA SAYS:

"If you love stuffed pork chops, you can make a pork loin imitate one quite nicely. Just cut your 12-ounce chunk into 4 equal slices, then slice each one almost all the way through (with your knife parallel to the counter) so they open up like a book. Stuff, close the "book," secure with toothpicks, and bake. Be sure to leave at least 1/2-inch along one side of each slice intact so the pieces stay together. Or, you can butterfly the roast by cutting it the same way as above, but opening it up, putting it between plastic wrap, and pounding it until it is very flat and thin, then filling it with stuffing and rolling it up, tying it with string and roasting it. Slice in 4 equal disks after baking for a delicious stuffed roast."

1 cup cornbread stuffing mix or crumbled homemade cornbread
2 teaspoons extra virgin olive oil
1/4 medium yellow or white onion chopped
1/4 sweet red bell pepper, seeded and chopped
1 4-oz. can diced green chili peppers, drained
1 teaspoon dried sage, crumbled

Dash of black or red cayenne pepper (or both if you like it zingy)
Add one of the following:
- 1 heaping tablespoon peeled and chopped small tart apple (like Granny Smith) drizzled with 1 teaspoon fresh lemon juice (to keep it from browning)
- 1 heaping tablespoon raisins or currants
- 1 heaping tablespoon fresh, frozen, or canned corn

1/4 to 1/2 cup low-fat, low-sodium chicken broth
12 oz. pork loin, cut into 4 equal slices, or butterflied and pounded flat

METHOD

1. Preheat oven to 375° F for 4 individual stuffed servings, or 325° F for a rolled roast. Put the cornbread crumbs into a large mixing bowl.
2. Spray a medium-sized nonstick skillet with nonstick cooking spray, then heat olive oil in the skillet over medium heat until you can smell the aroma of the oil. Add onion, red bell pepper, green chili peppers, sage, and black or red cayenne pepper. Sauté until onions are soft and translucent, about 8 minutes.
3. Remove from heat and stir in fruit or corn. Add to mixing bowl of cornbread crumbs and toss lightly. Drizzle with 1/4 cup low-fat, low-sodium chicken broth and toss until mixture looks moist but not mushy. Add more chicken broth if necessary.
4. Spray a shallow roasting pan with nonstick cooking spray. Stuff individual pork loin pieces with stuffing and secure with toothpicks, or spread stuffing over flattened pork loin roast and roll up, securing with string. Put stuffed pork loin into roasting pan and bake according to the following:
5. If you are baking individual loin pieces, bake for about 40 minutes or until pork is cooked through and juices run clear when meat is pierced.
6. If you are baking the rolled roast, insert a meat thermometer into the center of the roast and bake for about 1 hour or until the roast's internal temperature registers 155° F. Slice into 4 individual servings.

Both versions are delicious served with applesauce and a big salad.

(continued)

NUTRITIONAL INFORMATION PER SERVING

Calories 162
Total Fat 8.3 g
Saturated Fat 2.3 g
Unsaturated Fat 5.2 g
Cholesterol 35 mg
Sodium 315 mg
Carbohydrates 7.4 g
Protein 13.8 g
Food Exchange Value: 1/2 starch/bread, 1/2 vegetable, 3 medium-fat meat

Barbecue Pulled Pork Sandwiches

DONNA SAYS:

"This recipe practically begs to be made in the crockpot or crockery cooker because this method of cooking breaks down the meat, making it easy to pull apart with a fork for barbecue. Plus, cooking this way is so easy, it takes virtually no preparation time. You can easily double this recipe, then freeze half for next week. Barbecue sauce is usually fat-free, but check the label to make sure. And barbecue sauce does contain sugar, so go easy."

12-oz. pork loin
1/4 teaspoon salt
1/2 teaspoon black pepper
1 tablespoon chili powder
2 garlic cloves
1 large yellow onion
1 large red or green bell pepper
1/2 cup of your favorite barbecue sauce
1/2 cup orange juice
4 whole wheat sandwich buns

METHOD

1. Cut half-inch slits all over the pork loin. Rub the pork loin with the salt, pepper, and chili powder.

2. Peel and slice the garlic cloves, then insert garlic slices into the cuts in the pork.
3. Slice the onion. Slice and seed the peppers. Arrange onions and peppers on the bottom of the crockpot. Place the garlic-studded pork loin on top of the onions and peppers. Mix the barbecue sauce and orange juice until combined and pour over the roast and vegetables.
4. Cover crockpot and cook on low for about 8 hours or until the meat comes apart easily with a fork.
5. Remove meat from crockpot and put in a large bowl. With 2 forks, pull the pork loin into shreds. Spoon the sauce, onions, and peppers from the crockpot over the meat. Mix to combine and serve on buns. Delicious with a side of baked beans or butter beans and a salad.

Note: If you don't have a crockpot, you can make this recipe in the oven in a roasting pan, roasting at 325° F for about 90 minutes or until meat is fork-tender. Remove meat and let it stand for about ten minutes, then shred it and heat it in a saucepan with the sauce and vegetables from the roasting pan.

NUTRITIONAL INFORMATION PER SERVING

Calories 421
Total Fat 12.1 g
Saturated Fat 3.8 g
Unsaturated Fat 6.8 g
Cholesterol 69 mg
Sodium 642 mg
Carbohydrates 48.3 g
Protein 30.4 g
Food Exchange Value: 1 starch/bread, 1 fruit, 1 other carbohydrate, 3 medium-fat meat

Vegetable Pork Stir-Fry Medley

~~~~~~~~

DONNA SAYS:

"This recipe is easy to change according to whatever ingredients you have in the house and whatever mood strikes you. For a Caribbean flair, add some peeled sliced chunks of mango to the stir-fry just before serving. For stir-fry à la Jamaica, add a cubed sweet potato, a peeled and sliced plantain, a handful of dried apricots, and a dash of Jamaican jerk seasoning. For a Cajun twist, add a few boiled shrimp, a dash of cayenne pepper, and serve over yellow rice. Have fun with it! Let your creativity shine."

12-oz. pork loin, frozen then partially thawed (so you can slice it
    more easily)
1 tablespoon extra virgin olive oil
4 cups of your favorite vegetables (and fruits!) in whatever
    proportions you like:

        onions
        garlic
        bell peppers, any color
        hot peppers
        button mushrooms
        exotic mushrooms like portabello and shitake
        pea pods
        green beans
        broccoli
        cauliflower
        bok choy
        cabbage
        carrots
        celery
        corn
        baby corn
        hominy
        white potatoes
        sweet potatoes

    water chestnuts
    bamboo shoots
    white beans
    black eyed peas
dried fruit:
    1 tablespoon snipped pieces of dried apricots, prunes, or
       other dried fruit
    1 tablespoon raisins, golden raisins, currants, dried
       cranberries, or blueberries
    mango or papaya slices
    peach or nectarine slices
    apple slices
    mandarin oranges
    pear cubes
    peanuts, cashews, walnuts, or almonds (not more than 1
       tablespoon per serving)
herbs of your choice
1/4 cup apple juice
1 tablespoon low-sodium soy sauce
1 tablespoon cornstarch
2 cups hot cooked brown, yellow, white, or wild rice or noodles

METHOD

1. Slice the pork loin into thin strips, then julienne the strips so you have bite-sized strips of pork.
2. Spray a nonstick skillet or wok with cooking spray, then heat the olive oil in the skillet over medium-high heat until you can smell the oil's aroma.
3. Add pork to the skillet and sauté until cooked through, about 3 minutes. Move the pork to a plate.
4. Add vegetables and herbs to the skillet. Depending on which vegetables you choose, you may want to add the ones that require more cooking time first, but it's not really necessary. I usually gauge cooking time by the onions. When they are soft and translucent, and the other vegetables look bright and crisp, return the pork to the skillet and remove from heat.
5. In a small bowl, whisk apple juice, soy sauce, and cornstarch together until well combined.

(continued)

6. Return pork and vegetables to heat, add any fruits if using them, then pour apple juice mixture over the whole thing.
7. Mix and stir until sauce thickens, about 5 to 8 minutes. Serve immediately over rice or noodles.

NUTRITIONAL INFORMATION PER SERVING
Calories 390
Total Fat 14.2 g
Saturated Fat 4.05 g
Unsaturated Fat 8.8 g
Cholesterol 69 mg
Sodium 224 mg
Carbohydrates 37 g
Protein 30.5 g
Food Exchange Value: 2 fruit or vegetable, 1 starch/bread, 3 medium-fat meat

Marinated Beef Strips with Orange Brandy Sauce

DONNA SAYS:

"Beef doesn't have to be bad for you. Choose lean beef like a lean eye of round and cut it into thin slices. Marinate it to soften the fibers, then, after cooking, drizzle with a fancy sauce like this one (it only tastes fancy, it's easy to make). Beef's rich taste goes perfectly with a rich sauce like this. You'll end up with an elegant, gourmet meal that really satisfies."

Serves 4

MARINATED BEEF STRIPS
12-oz. eye of round steak or lean sirloin steak
1/2 teaspoon black pepper
1/2 cup orange juice
1/4 cup cider vinegar
4 cups lettuce leaves

METHOD

1. Put the beef in the freezer for about 1 hour, or until just partially frozen. This will make it easier to slice. Remove from the freezer and put the steak on a cutting board. Cut off any fat around the edges, and then slice as thin as you can.
2. Put the beef slices in a pie plate and sprinkle with pepper. Pour orange juice and vinegar over the beef, cover with plastic wrap, and put in the refrigerator. Allow to marinate for at least 2 hours, and up to 12 hours.
3. Spray a nonstick skillet with nonstick cooking spray. Remove beef slices from marinade and discard marinade. Heat beef over medium-high heat until cooked through, about 10 minutes, depending on how thin you made those slices.
4. Cover a platter with lettuce leaves and arrange beef slices over the lettuce. Drizzle with the Orange Brandy Sauce.

ORANGE BRANDY SAUCE

Note: If you don't want to use brandy, substitute apricot nectar and call this "Orange Apricot Sauce" instead.

1/4 cup orange juice concentrate
1/4 cup apple juice concentrate
1 tablespoon apricot brandy, apple brandy, or apricot nectar
1/4 cup apple juice
1 teaspoon grated orange peel
1 tablespoon cornstarch
1/4 cup water

METHOD

1. Combine orange juice concentrate, apple juice concentrate, brandy, apple juice, and grated orange peel in a nonstick sauce pan.
2. In a separate, small bowl or cup, whisk cornstarch into the water, then whisk the cornstarch mixture into the juice mixture.
3. Heat over medium heat, stirring constantly, until mixture begins to thicken and bubble. Allow to boil, stirring the whole time, for 1 full minute, then remove from heat.
4. Drizzle over warm beef strips. Cover and store any remaining sauce in the refrigerator. It's also good over cold meat.

(continued)

NUTRITIONAL INFORMATION PER SERVING
Calories 260
Total Fat 9 g
Saturated Fat 3.4 g
Unsaturated Fat 4 g
Cholesterol 66 mg
Sodium 67.6 mg
Carbohydrates 19 g
Protein 25 g
Food Exchange Value: 1 fruit, 1 vegetable, 3 lean meat

Honey Smoked Chicken

DONNA SAYS:
"It's fun to have a barbecue in the summer, but who needs all that fat in burgers and hot dogs? Try this grilled chicken breast instead, or just bake it in the oven if you don't feel like using the grill. The liquid smoke will still give it that smoky flavor."

Serves 8

1 cup dry white wine ("real" drinking wine tastes better than wine labeled "cooking wine") or 1 cup white grape juice
3 cloves garlic, peeled and minced
1 medium yellow onion, peeled and chopped
1/2 red bell pepper, cored, seeded, and chopped
1 teaspoon paprika
2 tablespoons honey
1/3 cup liquid smoke
Pepper to taste
8 skinless chicken breast halves (4 total breasts) on the bone

METHOD
1. In a food processor or blender, combine wine or juice, garlic, onion, red bell peppers, paprika, honey, liquid smoke, and pepper.

2. Spray your grill with a non-stick spray if using an electric grill, or if using a charcoal grill, wait until coals are white hot to spray. Or, preheat oven to 375° F and spray a roasting pan.

3. Rinse chicken breasts and pat dry with a paper towel. Arrange the chicken breasts on the grill (or in the pan) meat-side down, about 8 inches from the coals. Cook for 5 minutes. Flip chicken so meat side is up and cook for 5 more minutes.

4. Flip chicken again, meat side down, and brush generously with marinade. Cook for 5 more minutes. Flip again, brush remaining marinade over chicken pieces, and cook a final 5 minutes, or until chicken is cooked through and crispy.

NUTRITIONAL INFORMATION PER SERVING

Calories 196
Total Fat 5 g
Saturated Fat 1.1 g
Unsaturated Fat 3.3 g
Cholesterol 73 mg
Sodium 65.1 mg
Carbohydrate 9.5 g
Protein 27.2 g
Food Exchange Value: 2 vegetable, 3 1/2 very lean meat

Nutty Chicken Stir-Fry

~~~~~~~

DONNA SAYS:

"A stir-fry is a great way to get your vegetables and the flavor of meat without much fat. It's fun to make and the rice makes it filling. It's a lot better for you than fast-food take-out."

Serves 8

1 teaspoon sesame oil
2 boneless, skinless chicken breasts (4 halves), thinly sliced
1 small yellow or white onion, peeled and diced

(continued)

1 cup celery, thinly sliced

1 cup mushrooms, thinly sliced (portabello, shitake, straw or other
 Chinese mushrooms, or white button mushrooms)

1 5-oz. can bamboo shoots, drained

1/2 cup canned baby corn (the little tiny ears of corn), drained

1/2 cup canned water chestnuts, drained

1 tablespoon sherry

1 tablespoon low-sodium soy sauce

2 tablespoons cornstarch

1/2 teaspoon sugar

1/4 cup water

1 tablespoon sesame seeds

1/4 cup nuts: whole or sliced almonds, walnuts, cashews, peanuts,
 or a combination of your favorites

2 cups cooked brown or white rice

METHOD

1. Spray a large nonstick skillet or wok with nonstick cooking spray. Add
 half the sesame oil and heat over medium-high heat. Add chicken and
 cook, stirring constantly, for 5 minutes or until cooked through and
 golden brown. Remove chicken to a plate and set aside.

2. Remove wok or skillet from heat, spray with more cooking spray, add
 the remaining sesame oil, then add the onions, celery, and mushrooms.
 Cook, stirring constantly, for 5 minutes, or until onions are translucent
 and slightly brown.

3. To the wok, add the bamboo shoots, baby corn, water chestnuts, sherry,
 and soy sauce. Cook, stirring constantly, for an additional 5 minutes.

4. Whisk the cornstarch and sugar into the water in a small bowl. Slowly
 pour over the vegetable mixture in the wok. Stir to combine, then
 cover the skillet or wok and allow to cook without stirring for 5 minutes.

5. Uncover and add back the cooked chicken, and the sesame seeds and
 nuts. Stir to combine. Cook an additional 5 minutes to heat chicken
 through. Remove from heat and serve immediately over rice.

NUTRITIONAL INFORMATION PER SERVING

Calories 195

Total Fat 4.8 g

Saturated Fat .84 g

Unsaturated Fat 3.5 g

Cholesterol 36.6 mg

Sodium 161.8 mg

Carbohydrates 20.7 g

Protein 17 g

Food Exchange Value: 1 vegetable, 1 starch/bread, 2 very lean meat

Mustard Chicken with Collard Greens

DONNA SAYS:

"This tangy chicken tastes great with the mellow, sweet-yet-bitter taste of cooked collards, and you can't beat this meal for great nutrition!"

Serves 4

2 whole chicken breasts skinned, boned, and quartered

1/4 cup low sodium, fat-free chicken broth

1/4 cup brown mustard (like Dijon)

2 garlic cloves, peeled and minced

1 tablespoon cider vinegar

1 tablespoon brown sugar, packed

1 tablespoon dried tarragon, crushed

1 tablespoon canola oil

1 Vidalia onion (or other sweet onion), peeled and thinly sliced
   into rings

1 large bunch of collard greens, stemmed and coarsely chopped
   (about 4 cups)

METHOD

1. Spray a nonstick skillet with nonstick cooking spray. Put chicken breasts in pan and cook over medium heat until chicken breast is cooked through and golden brown, about 5 minutes on each side.
2. While chicken is cooking, whisk together chicken stock, mustard, garlic, vinegar, brown sugar, and tarragon in a small bowl until combined.

(continued)

Pour over chicken, lower heat to low, and cook an additional 5 minutes to warm the sauce.

3. In a soup pot or Dutch oven, heat canola oil over medium-high heat. Add onion and cook, stirring, until onion is translucent. Add half the collard greens, stir to combine with onions, and cover the pot. Allow to cook 5 minutes, or until collard greens cook down, wilting and reducing in size. Add the rest of the greens, stir to combine, then cover again for another 5 minutes or until all the collards have wilted and cooked down.

4. To serve, put collard greens on a platter and top with chicken. Drizzle remaining sauce over the chicken and greens.

NUTRITIONAL INFORMATION PER SERVING

Calories 234

Total Fat 8.2 g

Saturated Fat 1.2 g

Unsaturated Fat 6.6 g

Cholesterol 73.1 mg

Sodium 464 mg

Carbohydrates 10.8 g

Protein 29.6 g

Food Exchange Value: 2 vegetable, 3 1/2 very lean meat, 1 1/2 fat

Green-Chili Chicken Casserole

DONNA SAYS:

"This casserole is filling and very satisfying to eat, but it has hardly any fat. A salad and some fresh fruit are all this recipe needs to complete a meal."

Serves 10

2 pounds boneless, skinless chicken breast

2 cups lowfat, reduced sodium chicken broth, divided in half

2 cups water

1 cup cornmeal

1/4 cup flour

1 teaspoon low sodiume baking powder

1 teaspoon paprika

1/4 teaspoon black pepper

1 cup nonfat buttermilk

1 4-oz. can chopped green chilies

1 cup frozen corn

METHOD

1. Boil the chicken breasts in 1 cup chicken broth mixed with 2 cups water until tender and fully cooked, about 30 minutes. Remove chicken and pull into shreds on a cutting board, then spread over the bottom of a 13 x 9 baking pan.

2. Preheat the oven to 425° F.

3. Combine cornmeal, flour, baking powder, paprika, and pepper in a small bowl. Whisk in buttermilk and remaining 1 cup of chicken broth (undiluted). Add green chilies and corn and heat on low until simmering gently. Pour over chicken.

4. Bake for 1 hour or until bubbling and slightly browned.

NUTRITIONAL INFORMATION PER SERVING

Calories 246

Total Fat 4.5 g

Saturated Fat 1.3 g

Unsaturated Fat 2.4 g

Cholesterol 79 mg

Sodium 165 mg

Carbohydrates 19 g

Protein 32 g

Food Exchange Value: 1/2 starch/bread, 1/2 starchy vegetable, 3 1/2 very lean meat

Nutty Broccoli Toss

~~~~~~

DONNA SAYS:

"This is a delicious way to get your veggies. The small amounts of oil, cheese, and nuts add just enough fat to give this vegetable side dish great flavor, and it's all the kind of fat that, in small amounts, is good for your heart."

Serves 8

DRESSING
    1 teaspoon olive oil
    1/4 cup cider vinegar
    1 teaspoon cumin
    1 teaspoon Parmesan cheese
    Dash black pepper

SALAD
    2 cups steamed and cooled broccoli florets
    2 cups steamed and cooled cauliflower florets
    1/4 cup sliced green onions
    1 tablespoon sesame seeds
    1 tablespoon sunflower seeds, unsalted
    1 tablespoon slivered almonds
    1 tablespoon chopped walnuts

METHOD
1. Blend olive oil, vinegar, cumin, Parmesan cheese, and pepper in a small bowl with a wire whisk.
2. Combine broccoli, cauliflower, green onions, sesame seeds, sunflower seeds, almonds, and walnuts in a large bowl and toss lightly.
3. Pour dressing over salad mixture and toss lightly to coat. Sprinkle with sesame seeds.

NUTRITIONAL INFORMATION PER SERVING
    Calories 46
    Total Fat 3 g

Saturated Fat .35 g
Unsaturated Fat 1.8 g
Cholesterol .2 mg
Sodium 23.2 mg
Carbohydrates 4 g
Protein 2.3 g
Food Exchange Value: 1 vegetable, 1/2 fat

Better-Than-Fried Potatoes

DONNA SAYS:

"These potatoes are so delicious, warm and crispy and brown, that you'll never miss the high-fat version. Try substituting sweet potatoes for an absolutely delicious alternative. You'll have a hard time deciding which version you like best."

Serves 8

4 baking potatoes or sweet potatoes, scrubbed, eyes removed
Dried paprika, oregano, thyme, or other favorite spice (but just use one), about 1 tablespoon or a little more. Try cinnamon for sweet potatoes.

METHOD
1. Preheat oven to 400° F.
2. Cut potatoes into 1/4-inch slices or 1/4-inch-thick strips, depending on whether you want a chip shape or a French-fry shape.
3. Spray a baking sheet with the butter-flavored cooking spray, then place potato pieces on the sheet. Spray potatoes, then sprinkle on your herb or spice of choice.
4. Bake for 30 minutes, or until potatoes are nicely browned and slightly crisp. Serve warm with ketchup, or try these with the Herb Garden Dip (great with baking potatoes) or the Caribbean Chutney (great with sweet potatoes).

(continued)

NUTRITIONAL INFORMATION PER SERVING

Calories 69
Total Fat .27 g
Saturated Fat .05 g
Unsaturated Fat .12 g
Cholesterol 0
Sodium 5.29 mg
Carbohydrates 15.5 g
Protein 1.9 g
Food Exchange Value: 1 starchy vegetable

Steamed Spring Veggies

DONNA SAYS:

"This seems like an old stand-by when it comes to vegetable side dishes, but you'll be surprised how much better it tastes when you make it at home than when you cook up a bag of the frozen stuff from the store. It's a great way to make use of early spring produce, and during other times of year, you can make this with pea pods and fresh carrots, or even frozen peas. (You can always buy fresh carrots.) This recipe has just a little bit of butter to make it really flavorful, but not so much that it adds a lot of fat."

Serves 6

1 cup freshly shelled baby green peas (or 2 cups frozen baby peas)
1 cup baby carrots, quartered the long way to make matchsticks
1 cup pencil-thin asparagus, tough ends removed, cut into 1-inch
   pieces
1 teaspoon butter
1 tablespoon fresh dill or 1 teaspoon dried dill

METHOD

1. Combine peas, carrots, and asparagus in a steamer basket and place over boiling water. Steam until carrots are tender, about 10 minutes.
2. Put vegetable mixture into a bowl. Toss with butter and dill.
3. Serve warm.

NUTRITIONAL INFORMATION PER SERVING

Calories 37.6

Total Fat .84 g

Saturated Fat .45 g

Unsaturated Fat .31 g

Cholesterol 1.83 mg

Sodium 12.2 mg

Carbohydrate 5.7 g

Protein 2.1 g

Food Exchange Value: 1 vegetable

Lemon-Butter Broccoli Florets

DONNA SAYS:

"If you think you don't like broccoli, maybe you aren't cooking it in an interesting way. Broccoli can be bland or even terrible when overcooked, but steamed until tender but crisp and flavored just right, it's one of the most delicious vegetable side dishes you can make. It's also one of the most nutrient-packed vegetables you can find, so it's a great addition to anyone's diet. I say try to eat some broccoli at least once a week!"

Serves 8

4 cups broccoli florets

1 lemon

1 teaspoon real butter

METHOD

1. Steam broccoli in a steamer basket over boiling water until bright green and crisp-tender. Do not overcook! Keep an eye on it.
2. Grate the zest (the yellow part) from the lemon and set aside. Squeeze the juice from the lemon and set aside.
3. Remove florets from steamer and put in a large bowl. Immediately toss with 1 teaspoon butter. Sprinkle with grated lemon zest and lemon juice.
4. Toss and serve immediately.

(continued)

NUTRITIONAL INFORMATION PER SERVING

Calories 23.3
Total Fat .53 g
Saturated Fat .32 g
Unsaturated Fat .18 g
Cholesterol 1.4 mg
Sodium 18.7 mg
Carbohydrates 3.34 mg
Protein 1.42 g
Food Exchange Value: 1 vegetable

Winter Vegetable Mix

~~~~~~~

DONNA SAYS:

"Baby spring vegetables are delicious, but so are the heartier root vegetables of winter. Try this recipe when the weather gets cold. It's nutritious and warming."

Serves 10

1 baking potato, scrubbed and diced (put diced potato into a bowl
   of ice water to keep it from discoloring)
1 cup frozen lima beans
1 cup carrots, scrubbed and sliced
1 cup parsnip, rutabaga, or kohlrabi, peeled and cubed
1 cup butternut or acorn squash, peeled and cubed
1 cup frozen green beans
1 cup frozen green peas
1 15- or 16-oz. can light red kidney beans or great northern beans,
   drained and rinsed
1 tablespoon cumin
1 teaspoon each oregano and basil
1/2 teaspoon thyme
Pinch of allspice

METHOD

1. Combine all ingredients in a soup pot, Dutch oven, or a crockpot. Fill pot with just enough water to cover or, if using the crockpot, don't add any water but sprinkle the spices over the veggies.
2. For the soup pot or Dutch oven, bring water to a boil, then reduce heat, cover, and simmer until potatoes are fork-tender and frozen veggies are thoroughly cooked, about 40 minutes. Add more water during cooking if necessary.
3. If using a crockpot, cook on low for 8 to 10 hours.
4. To serve, drain veggies and reserve juices for soup or other vegetable stock use (refrigerate and use within 1 week or freeze). Or, serve as a vegetarian main course with rice, and ladle some of the vegetable juices over the rice. Or serve as a winter vegetable soup. Whichever way you like it!

NUTRITIONAL INFORMATION PER SERVING

Calories 130
Total Fat .6 g
Saturated Fat .05 g
Unsaturated Fat .12 g
Cholesterol 0
Sodium 108 mg
Carbohydrates 25.9 g
Protein 6.4 g
Food Exchange Value: 1 starchy vegetable, 2 vegetable

Creamy Cornbread Muffins

~~~~~~

DONNA SAYS:

"Cornbread muffins are good any time of day—for breakfast, for lunch, as a side dish for dinner, or as a healthy and hearty snack. Some versions are high in fat, but this one is both moist and flavorful without all the butter or lard you find in some recipes. Using creamed corn and sour cream keeps these low in fat."

Serves 12

1 cup sifted flour
1cup yellow cornmeal
2 1/2 teaspoons low sodium baking powder
1 egg plus 2 egg whites
1/2 cup nonfat sour cream
1/4 cup canola oil or corn oil
2 tablespoons honey
1 16-oz. can creamed corn (make sure it contains no fat)
1/2 cup frozen whole corn kernels
optional: 1 tablespoon diced jalapeno peppers (if you like it spicy)
    or green chilies (if you like it kind of spicy)

METHOD

1. Preheat oven to 425° F.
2. Sift together flour, corn meal, and baking powder in a large bowl.
3. Add egg, egg whites, sour cream, oil, honey, and creamed corn. Stir lightly with a fork until just mixed.
4. Lightly fold in frozen corn and optional peppers or chilies.
5. Spray a muffin tin with nonstick cooking spray and fill each tin about 2/3 full of batter.
6. Bake about 30 minutes or until light golden brown.

NUTRITIONAL INFORMATION PER SERVING

Calories 178
Total Fat 4.2 g

Saturated Fat .51 g

Unsaturated Fat 4.7 g

Cholesterol 15.6 mg

Sodium 32.9 mg

Carbohydrates 29 g

Protein 4.22 g

Food Exchange Value: 1 starch/bread, 1 starchy vegetable

Fresh Berry Country Waffles

DONNA SAYS:

"Everybody loves waffles for breakfast, but those frozen ones from the store just aren't the same as homemade. This version uses healthy whole wheat flour for fiber and fresh berries. Try it in the summertime, changing berries according to what you can find fresh at the local market."

Serves 8

3 tablespoons canola oil

1 tablespoon packed brown sugar

2 cups nonfat buttermilk

1 cup whole wheat flour

1 cup all purpose flour

2 teaspoons low sodium baking powder

1 1/2 teaspoons grated orange peel

3 egg whites

1 cup fresh blueberries (or, frozen unsweetened berries)

METHOD

1. In a large bowl, whisk together the canola oil and brown sugar until well combined. Whisk in buttermilk.
2. In a medium bowl, whisk wheat flour, white flour, baking powder, and grated orange peel together, then lightly whisk the flour mixture into the milk mixture.
3. Using an electric mixer, beat egg whites until soft peaks form.
4. Fold egg whites and blueberries lightly into the batter.

(continued)

5. Spray waffle iron with nonstick cooking spray, pour batter in according to the manufacturer's directions for your waffle maker, and cook until golden brown.

NUTRITIONAL INFORMATION PER SERVING

Calories 206
Total Fat 7.4 g
Saturated Fat .83 g
Unsaturated Fat 5.05 g
Cholesterol 3.75 mg
Sodium 90 mg
Carbohydrates 31 g
Protein 7.4 g
Food Exchange Value: 1 bread, 1 milk, 1/2 fruit, 1/2 very lean meat

Chai-Spiced Peach Mousse

DONNA SAYS:

"Your family will love the rich, creamy taste and smooth texture of this frozen fruit mousse, and the exotic flavor of chai spices—from the Indian tea drink that has become so popular in coffee houses—blends in just the right way with the bananas. No refined sugar here—only the fruit's natural sugar for sweetness. No cream."

Serves 6

2 1/2 cups frozen peach slices (pit and slice fresh peaches, wrap in a heavy freezer bag, and freeze overnight or buy a bag of frozen peaches)
1/2 cup part-skim ricotta cheese
1/2 cup nonfat buttermilk
1 teaspoon vanilla extract
1 1/2 teaspoons masala (the Indian spice mixture), or if you can't find masala, use 1 teaspoon cinnamon, 1/4 teaspoon cardamom, 1/4 teaspoon ground nutmeg, and a dash of ground cloves

GARNISH

cinnamon sticks, fresh banana slices, ground cinnamon

METHOD

1. Put all ingredients in a food processor fitted with a steel blade or a blender (the food processor works best for this one—you may need to add a little additional buttermilk or some skim milk if your blender isn't very heavy-duty).
2. Process or blend until well combined, smooth, and creamy, about 1–2 minutes.
3. Serve immediately in glass dessert dishes or teacups, garnished with a cinnamon stick and a couple of sliced bananas sprinkled with cinnamon.

MORE MOUSSE FLAVORS

- Don't care for peaches, or can't find ripe ones? Try ripe bananas, strawberries, apricots, Bing cherries, or any really ripe fruit that mashes well. You'll need about 2 1/2 cups of fresh or frozen fruit or about 6 ripe, frozen bananas to mash. If you are using pre-packaged frozen fruit, look for brands that have no added sugar and that are not packed in syrup.
- Who says you need to use just one kind of fruit? Try a banana-strawberry blend, a peach-apricot blend, a blackberry-blueberry blend. Whatever lights your taste buds up. Adjust spices if you don't like the chai spices—cinnamon and vanilla alone are great.

NUTRITIONAL INFORMATION PER SERVING

Calories 71
Total fat 2 g
Saturated fat 1.2 g
Unsaturated fat .65 g
Cholesterol 7.6 mg
Sodium 47.8 mg
Carbohydrates 10.6 g
Protein 3.6 g
Food Exchange Value: 1/2 fruit, 1/2 milk

Chocolate Spice Cake with Dark Chocolate Glaze

~~~~~~~

DONNA SAYS:

"Can you make a great tasting cake without sugar? Well, almost! This chocolate spice cake gets most of its sweetness from fruit, with just a little sugar, and it's virtually fat free. The trick is to keep your serving size down when it comes to the sweet stuff. Divide the cake into 12 pieces, give everyone at the table one piece, and send the rest home with guests or take it to the neighbors."

Serves 12

2 1/2 cups all purpose flour
1/3 cup brown sugar, packed
1/2 cup cocoa powder
1 teaspoon low sodium baking powder
1/2 teaspoon baking soda
1 tablespoon ground cinnamon
1 teaspoon ground ginger
1/2 teaspoon ground nutmeg
2 egg whites
1 8-oz. carton (or 1 cup) plain nonfat yogurt
1 cup canned pumpkin puree (not pumpkin pie filling)
1 cup prune juice (the kind that is 100% juice)
1/4 cup unsweetened black coffee, brewed or prepared instant

METHOD
1. Pre-heat oven to 350° F. Spray a 9x13 cake pan or a standard-sized Bundt pan with nonstick cooking spray.
2. In a medium bowl combine flour, sugar, cocoa powder, baking powder, baking soda, and spices. Set aside.
3. In a large bowl, combine egg whites, yogurt, pumpkin, prune juice, and coffee. Beat at medium speed until well combined.
4. Add 1/3 of the flour mixture to the batter and beat on low for 1 minute. Add 1/2 the yogurt and beat 1 minute. Repeat, alternating 1/3 flour mixture and the other half of the yogurt, until well combined.

5. Pour the batter into the pan and bake for 45 minutes or until a toothpick inserted into the center comes out clean.
6. Cool on wire rack in pan. If using a Bundt pan, after 10 minutes carefully turn out onto a plate.
7. Drizzle with Dark Chocolate Glaze.

DARK CHOCOLATE GLAZE

This glaze can taste spicy-fruity if you use the orange juice, or like Mexican chocolate (it's that touch of cinnamon that does the trick) if you use the coffee. Both versions are tasty and complement the cake, so try them both at separate, special occasions.

   1/4 cup cocoa
   2 tablespoons confectioner's (powdered) sugar
   1/4 teaspoon cinnamon
   2 tablespoons (or a little more or less, to achieve the right consistency) orange juice or black coffee, brewed or prepared instant

Combine cocoa, sugar, and cinnamon in a small bowl. Mix in orange juice or coffee, one tablespoon at a time, until glaze is thick but pourable.

NUTRITIONAL INFORMATION PER SERVING
   Calories 180
   Total Fat .86 g
   Saturated Fat .36 g
   Unsaturated Fat .39 g
   Cholesterol .42 mg
   Sodium 79 mg
   Carbohydrates 37.5 g
   Protein 5.8 g
   Food Exchange Value: 1 fruit, 1 starch/bread, 1/2 milk

Pear Tofu Cheesecake Amandine

~~~~~~~

DONNA SAYS:

"This cheesecake tastes rich and creamy. You won't believe it's got tofu instead of cream cheese!"

Serves 8

3 tablespoons ground almonds
3 tablespoons barley nugget cereal (like Grape Nuts)
4 egg whites
1/4 cup all-purpose flour
1 pound firm tofu
1/2 cup sugar
1 teaspoon almond extract
1 teaspoon vanilla extract
8 oz. nonfat sour cream
2 cups sliced fresh or drained canned pears
1/2 teaspoon coriander
1 tablespoon sliced almonds

METHOD

1. Preheat oven to 400° F. Spray a 9-inch springform pan with non-stick cooking spray.
2. Heat ground almonds and cereal in a dry skillet over medium-high heat for about 5 minutes or until golden. Sprinkle ground almonds over the bottom of the cake pan.
3. Put egg whites, flour, tofu, sugar, almond extract, and vanilla extract into a food processor fitted with a steel blade or a blender. Process or blend until smooth and creamy, about 2–3 minutes, scraping down the sides once or twice.
4. Pour mixture in springform pan and bake for 10 minutes.
5. Remove cheesecake and lower oven heat to 225° F. Spread sour cream over the top and bake for an additional 80 minutes.
6. Remove from oven and let cool for 10 minutes. Loosen sides of cheesecake with a knife and release the side of the pan. Let cool for 1 hour, then refrigerate overnight.

7. To serve, puree pears in a blender or food processor with the coriander. Pour about 1/4 cup of pear puree on a plate, top with a slice of cheesecake, and sprinkle a few sliced almonds on top.

NUTRITIONAL INFORMATION PER SERVING

Calories 234

Total Fat 7.3 g

Saturated Fat .88 g

Unsaturated Fat 5.7 g

Cholesterol 0

Sodium 90 mg

Carbohydrates 30.3 g

Protein 13.4 g

Food Exchange Value: 1 fruit, 1 lean meat, 1 medium-fat meat, 1/2 milk

Appendix A

~~~~~~

Recipe Substitutions: What Goes with What?

Sometimes you really want to make a recipe but find you don't have all the right ingredients. Running to the store is not an option, or perhaps you haven't been able to find the ingredient. In a pinch, you can substitute one ingredient for another—inventive food artists do it all the time! Remember that trying new flavors, textures, and taste combinations is part of the fun of exploring your Menu for Life. If you like something, then great! If you don't care for a particular ingredient, try something else. Here are some common ingredient substitutions. Enjoy discovering what really works for you and keeps your family coming back for more healthful, adventurous, creative meals!

HERBS AND SPICES

Most herbs and spices are easy to substitute for similar flavors. You also can mix your own spice blends instead of buying pre-mixed blends at the grocery store that may be too high in sodium. Making your own spice blends also allows you to adjust the amounts of all the individual spices to suit your tastes. Who says you have to use someone else's blend? Make it your own.

Herb or Spice	Amount	Substitute	Amount
Herbs, fresh	1 tablespoon	herbs, dried	1 teaspoon
Herbs, dried	1 teaspoon	herbs, ground	1/2 teaspoon
Allspice	1 teaspoon	*Blend of:*	
		cinnamon	1/2 teaspoon
		nutmeg	1/4 teaspoon
		ground cloves	1/4 teaspoon
Aniseed	Any amount	fennel seed	equal amount
Apple pie spice	1 teaspoon	*Blend of:*	
		cinnamon	1/2 teaspoon
		nutmeg	1/4 teaspoon
		allspice	1/8 teaspoon
		ginger	1/8 teaspoon
		ground cloves	dash
Basil	Any amount	oregano or thyme	equal amount
Cajun spice	1 tablespoon	*Blend of:*	
		garlic powder	1/2 teaspoon
		onion powder	1/2 teaspoon
		black pepper	1/2 teaspoon
		white pepper	1/2 teaspoon
		cayenne or	
		ground red pepper	1/2 teaspoon
		paprika	1/2 teaspoon
Cardamom	Any amount	Ginger	equal amount
Cayenne pepper	1/4 teaspoon	bottled hot pepper	
		sauce or	1/4 teaspoon
		black pepper	1/4 teaspoon
Chervil	Any amount	tarragon or parsley	equal amount
Chili powder	1 tablespoon	*Blend of:*	
		cumin	2 teaspoons
		paprika	1/2 teaspoon
		oregano	1/2 teaspoon
		cayenne pepper or	dash
		bottled hot pepper	
		sauce	
Chives, fresh chopped	1 tablespoon	chopped: green	1 tablespoon
		onions or onions	
		or leeks	
Cilantro	Any amount	parsley or Italian	equal amount
		parsley	
Cinnamon, ground	1 teaspoon	nutmeg or allspice	1/4 teaspoon
Cumin	Any amount	chili powder	equal amount
Garlic	1 clove	garlic powder or	1/2 teaspoon
		minced garlic	1 teaspoon
Ginger, fresh grated	1 tablespoon	powdered ginger	1/2 teaspoon
Ginger, powdered	Any amount	allspice or	equal amount
		cinnamon or mace	
		or nutmeg	

Herb or Spice	Amount	Substitute	Amount
Italian seasoning, dried	1 teaspoon	*Blend of:*	
		basil	1/4 teaspoon
		oregano	1/4 teaspoon
		rosemary	1/4 teaspoon
		marjoram	1/4 teaspoon
Mace	Any amount	allspice or cinnamon or ginger or nutmeg	equal amount
Marjoram	Any amount	basil or savory or thyme	equal amount
Mint	Any amount	rosemary	equal amount
Mustard	1 teaspoon dry	prepared mustard	1 tablespoon
Nutmeg	Any amount	cinnamon or ginger or mace	equal amount
Oregano	Any amount	basil or thyme	equal amount
Parsley	Any amount	chervil or cilantro or Italian parsley	equal amount
Poultry seasoning	1 teaspoon	*Blend of:*	
		ground sage	1/2 teaspoon
		thyme	1/4 teaspoon
		marjoram	1/4 teaspoon
		black pepper	dash
Pumpkin pie spice	1 teaspoon	*Blend of:*	
		cinnamon	1/2 teaspoon
		ginger	1/4 teaspoon
		allspice	1/8 teaspoon
		nutmeg	1/8 teaspoon
Rosemary	any amount	thyme or tarragon or savory	equal amount
Saffron	any amount	turmeric	equal amount
Sage	any amount	poultry seasoning or savory or marjoram or rosemary	equal amount
Savory	any amount	thyme or marjoram or sage	equal amount
Tarragon	any amount	chervil or fennel seed or aniseed	equal amount
Thyme	any amount	basil or marjoram or oregano or savory	equal amount

SPICES TO USE WITH YOUR FAVORITE MEATS, POULTRY, AND SEAFOOD

Spices and seasonings add flavor to your favorite meats, poultry, and seafood. Remember that a little goes a long way. Typically, between one and four different herbs or spices is enough for most recipes, unless the recipe has been tested and says otherwise. Of course, it never hurts to experiment!

WITH THIS	TRY UP TO FOUR OF THESE
Beef	Garlic, cracked black pepper, chili powder, garlic and onion powder, oregano, parsley, ginger, sesame seeds, fresh basil, thyme, rosemary, red pepper flakes, bay leaf. For a Greek flavor, try cinnamon, cumin, allspice, and cocoa powder.
Pork	Garlic, rosemary, fennel, black and red pepper, cinnamon, lemon juice, nutmeg, cloves, sage, thyme, allspice, oregano.
Chicken	Sage, garlic, thyme, oregano, basil, savory, marjoram, tarragon, bay leaves, black and red pepper. For more exotic tastes, try curry powder, chili powder, ginger, cinnamon, cloves, nutmeg, allspice, coriander.
Turkey	Sage, basil, oregano, parsley, rosemary, black and red pepper. For a more exotic taste, try cinnamon, cocoa powder, chili powder, curry powder.
Light fish	Light, delicate herbs like parsley, dill, chervil, basil, thyme, fennel, lemon.
Fatty fish	Bolder herbs and spices like oregano, mint, chili powder, black and red pepper, bay leaves, fresh basil, cumin, coriander, cinnamon, fresh cilantro, and onion and garlic powder.
Shellfish	Lemon, pepper, garlic, paprika, basil, thyme, marjoram, parsley, curry powder, chili powder, cumin, ginger.

MEAT, POULTRY, AND SEAFOOD

Red meat, white meat, dark meat, shellfish, ocean fish . . . how do you know which is best? It seems every day we hear in the news what we should eat or what we shouldn't eat, but the key is to eat moderate portion sizes. Keep your portion size to three ounces cooked and you can enjoy most any kind of meat, poultry, or seafood for your meal. But what if you want to make a recipe and you don't have the right kind of meat? You can substitute most kinds of meat, poultry, and seafood for each other in many different dishes.

Beef and pork	Stick with cuts that have "loin" or "round" in the names, like sirloin, eye of round, round steak, pork loin, or tenderloin. These are the leanest. Any of these can be substituted for each other in recipes.
	Beef and pork are easy to switch in recipes. Pork tends to be a little lighter in color and flavor but both can be lean and are full of protein. Try some of your favorite beef recipes with pork, and pork recipes with beef.
Ground beef	Substitute ground turkey breast for ground beef for a lighter flavor and less fat. Chili, tacos, burgers, meatloaf, all the old standards you've always made with ground beef taste great made with ground turkey.
	Increase the spices by just a little to add extra hearty flavor to your ground turkey. If you aren't sure what spices to use, try oregano, basil, cumin, chili powder, paprika, and/or thyme to make ground turkey taste even more interesting. Or, try a dash of cinnamon in your ground turkey chili to give it a Greek flavor.
Poultry	Just as you can usually switch beef and pork in recipes with good results, you can almost always switch chicken and turkey.
	Stick to the white breast meat most of the time for both chicken and turkey for the lowest fat and highest protein.
	A chicken oriental stir-fry will have a different taste with turkey, but it will still be good. Barbecued turkey breast is a nice change from chicken.
Seafood	When it comes to seafood, you've got your light fish that are low in fat and somewhat delicate, good for cooking as a fillet and serving with vegetables or using in recipes.
	You've also got your fatty cold-water fish from cold deep water that contain the good kind of fat that helps to lower that "bad" cholesterol. These fatty fish are good for grilling and their firmer texture helps hold them together better for steaks. Then, of course, you've got your shellfish. Substitute any fish for any other in the same category for good results.
Low-fat fish	Atlantic pollock, Pacific pollock, blackfish, carp, catfish, cod, sole, grouper, haddock, halibut, bass, orange roughy, walleye, pike, ocean perch, tilapia, tilefish.
High-fat fish	Salmon, tuna (Albacore, Bluefin, Yellowfin), herring, bluefish, mackerel, sardines, red snapper, striped bass (rockfish), swordfish.

(continued)

Shellfish: shrimp, crawfish, scallops, clams, mussels, oysters, crabs, lobsters, octopus, and squid	Shrimp, crawfish, and scallops, are all easily interchangeable in any dish, but bite-sized chunks of snow crab or lobster can also stand in.
	Mussels and softshell crabs are interchangeable in most recipes.
	Oysters and hardshell clams are interchangeable in most recipes.
	Squid, octopus, and cuttlefish are interchangeable in most recipes.

VEGETABLES AND FRUITS

Most of us could stand to eat more vegetables and fruits, but sometimes it is hard to know what to cook or what to do with them. Soups, stews, chilis, stir frys, rice dishes, pasta, are all good with different combinations of vegetables. The trick is not to use *too* many or the flavor gets too complicated. Stick to about three to five different vegetables in combination dishes, or two vegetable side dishes with meat plus a salad. Try to include at least one root vegetable, one leafy green vegetable, one bright red, yellow, or orange vegetable (lots of root vegetables also qualify in this category), and one other kind of vegetable in your dinner, with some fruit at the end. That will give you variety in both taste and nutrition, and it will make your plate look more interesting too. Here are some examples of the different types of vegetables.

Root vegetables	Carrots, radishes, turnips, kohlrabi, rutabagas, parsnips, potatoes, sweet potatoes, yams, beets
Dark leafy greens	Collard greens, kale, mustard greens, spinach, escarole, watercress, leaf lettuces (not iceberg lettuce), broccoli, Brussels sprouts
Red, orange, and yellow vegetables	Red, yellow, and orange bell peppers, tomatoes, carrots, sweet potatoes, yams, acorn squash, butternut squash, beets
Other healthy vegetables	Green beans, green peas, okra, onions, garlic, cauliflower, corn, eggplant, mushrooms, pea pods, green and red cabbage, asparagus, spaghetti squash, artichoke
Fruits	In most recipes, you can substitute any berries for each other: strawberries, blueberries, blackberries, red and black raspberries.
	Gooseberries can stand in for rhubarb, and vice versa.
	Don't use melons or kiwi in cooked fruit recipes. They won't taste very good.
	Ripe bananas make baked recipes creamier.
	In most baked recipes, you can substitute ripe mashed bananas, pumpkin puree, or applesauce for some or all of the fat and still get a moist result.

ALREADY IN THE KITCHEN SUBSTITUTION LIST

For those times when you just plain run into trouble because you are out of sugar or tomato sauce or baking powder, these substitutions can bail you out.

ITEM	AMOUNT	YOU CAN REPLACE WITH	AMOUNT
Baking powder	1 teaspoon	*Blend of:*	
		baking soda	1/4 teaspoon
		cream of tartar	1/2 teaspoon
Buttermilk, nonfat	1 cup	plain nonfat yogurt or	1 cup
		nonfat sour cream or	1 cup
		lemon juice or vinegar	1 tablespoon
		plus skim milk	enough to make 1 cup
Cocoa	1/2 cup	sweet chocolate (and decrease butter or oil in the recipe by 1 tablespoon per 2 ounces)	2 ounces
Cornstarch	1 tablespoon	all-purpose flour	2 tablespoons
Egg	1 large	egg whites or	2
		egg substitute	1/4 cup
Flour	1 cup	whole wheat flour plus	1/2 cup
		all-purpose flour	1/2 cup
Honey	1 cup	white sugar plus	1 1/4 cup
		water or	1/4 cup
		molasses	1 cup
Lemon juice	1 teaspoon	Vinegar	1/2 teaspoon
Milk, skim	1 cup	evaporated skim milk plus	1/2 cup
		water or	1/2 cup
		nonfat dry milk powder	1/3 cup
		plus water	1 cup
Mushrooms, fresh	16 ounces	canned mushrooms, drained	10-ounce can
Nonfat sour cream	1 cup	nonfat buttermilk or	1 cup
		plain nonfat yogurt or	1 cup
		skim milk plus	1 cup
		lemon juice (allow to sit for 5 minutes at room temperature)	1 teaspoon
Onion	1 medium	instant minced onion or	2 tablespoons
		onion powder	1 tablespoon
Orange	1 medium	orange juice	1/2 cup

(continued)

Item	Amount	You Can Replace With	Amount
Peppers, bell		green, yellow, and red can be interchanged	
Sugar, brown	1 cup	molasses	2 tablespoons
Sugar, white	1 cup	powdered sugar or	1 cup (or 2 cups sifted)
		packed brown sugar or	1 cup
		corn syrup or	1 cup
		honey	1 cup
			(when using corn syrup or honey, decrease other liquids in recipe by 1/4 cup per 1 cup of liquid sweetener)
Tomato juice	1 cup	tomato sauce plus	1/2 cup
		water	1/2 cup
Tomato sauce (no sodium)	2 cups	tomato paste plus	3/4 cup
		water	1 cup water
Tomatoes, fresh, chopped	2 cups	canned tomatoes, drained (no sodium)	16-ounce can
Yogurt, plain nonfat	1 cup	nonfat buttermilk or	1 cup
		nonfat sour cream or	1 cup
		cottage cheese plus	1 cup
		lemon juice or vinegar blended on high until no curds remain	1 teaspoon

Substitutions to Reduce Fat, Sodium, and Calories in Favorite Recipes

Just follow these additional tips for updating, substituting, and changing things around to reduce fat, sodium, and calories without sacrificing taste.

Instead of This	Use This
Butter	Replace some or all of the butter with equal amounts of applesauce, mashed bananas, canned pumpkin puree (not pumpkin pie mix), or apple butter.
Dairy products	You can almost always substitute the whole fat types of milk, yogurt, and cheese with lowfat or nonfat varieties like skim milk, nonfat yogurt, and lowfat or nonfat cheese. You can also replace regular milk with soy milk.
Flour	Replace all white flour with half white, half whole wheat flour to add more nutrients and fiber in your baked goods.

Instead of This	Use This
Sugar	It's easy to replace white sugar with brown sugar or honey, but these options have just as many calories.
	Fruit juice concentrates are more nutritious but they are tough to substitute because they throw off the wet ingredient/dry ingredient ratio in your recipes, so you may have to experiment a little bit.
	Or, just simply try reducing the sugar by about half and adding fruit purée from very ripe fruit, or even baby food made from fruit (the kind without added sugar or tapioca). Baby food can be great in baking!
	For example, if a cake recipe calls for 1 cup of sugar, try using 1/2 cup white sugar and 1/2 cup baby food applesauce, peaches, or prunes. If your favorite cookie recipe uses 3/4 cup brown sugar, try using about 1/3 cup brown sugar and one mashed very ripe banana.

In Salads

Most dressings are high in fat, and nonfat dressings you buy in the store can be less than tasty. But when you make your own dressing, you don't have to use very much, if any, oil. Instead, mix fruit juices, nonfat yogurt, or buttermilk with a little vinegar and some fresh herbs. And make salads bigger and the fattening parts of the meal smaller! Have two cups of salad with nonfat dressing and less of the dishes that contain a lot of meat and cheese.

Instead of This	Try This
Meat and cheese	You can usually reduce the meat in a main course recipe and replace it, cup for cup, with chopped vegetables. Vegetables with a meaty texture like fresh chopped tomatoes, mushrooms, or even tofu crumbles that taste and look a lot like ground meat, make substitution easy.
	You can also usually reduce the cheese or use lowfat or nonfat cheese or even, again, tofu or soy cheese.
Oils	The oils used for sautéing can easily be replaced with stock or broth, or be eliminated altogether if you cook in a good nonstick skillet and use non-stick cooking spray. Just be sure to go light on the cooking spray and treat your nonstick cookware gently! Always wash it right away with a soft wash cloth only—no scrubbers please! You usually don't even need to use soap. Only use wooden or soft-edged plastic spoons or spatulas when cooking with nonstick cookware.

INSTEAD OF THIS	TRY THIS
Sandwiches	Sandwiches can make a great meal, unless you load them up with mayonnaise, butter, and lots of fatty meats and cheeses.
	Instead, make sandwiches with no more than 3 ounces of lean meat and lowfat or nonfat cheese in total, then use nonfat or lowfat mayonnaise and other, non-fat condiments like mustard, and lots of vegetables like leafy green lettuces, tomato slices, onion slices, sliced mushrooms, and green pepper rings.

IN VEGETABLES

Vegetables taste much better and are more nutritious when they are still a bit crunchy, so steaming is your best option. Or cook them with just a little water in a covered casserole in the microwave. Once vegetables are done, serve them quickly, and avoid drowning them in butter or oil. A splash of lemon juice, a few drops of olive oil, or a spritz of butter-flavored nonstick cooking spray with some fresh snipped herbs and maybe a few red pepper flakes make vegetables taste fresh, flavorful, and delicious.

Appendix B

~~~~~~~~

Take Any Recipe
and Make It Your Own

We all have those recipes that are family favorites, whether they are foods you remember from childhood or dishes you discovered once you were running your own kitchen. They are the meals that everybody just loves, the foods we take comfort in eating. The trouble is that lots of our beloved comfort foods are full of fat, sodium, or sugar. When you are losing weight and getting healthy, you may think many of your favorite foods will have to stay in the "no" column and you will have to give them up for good. Not so! You *can* have your macaroni and cheese, lasagna, fried fish, or even dessert. All you have to do is to learn to cook these favorites in a way that ups their nutrient density and lowers the fat, sodium, and empty calories.

Let's look at typical meal of lasagna, made with lots of meat and plenty of cheese, with some buttery garlic bread on the side. We'll show you how to take a traditional high-fat, high-sodium recipe and convert it into a Menu for Life comfort food favorite! Here are the ingredients for lasagna and buttery garlic bread the way you may be used to making them now:

High-Fat, Empty Calorie Lasagna

~~~~~~~~

1 pound ground beef or pork sausage
1 large onion, chopped
1 clove garlic, minced
1 8-oz. can tomato sauce
1 6-oz. can tomato paste
1 tablespoon Italian seasoning
6 dried lasagna noodles
1 beaten egg
16-oz. carton creamy cottage cheese
1/3 cup grated Romano cheese
8 oz. shredded mozzarella cheese
Parmesan cheese for garnish

High-Fat, High-Sodium Garlic Bread

~~~~~~~~

1 loaf Italian bread cut into 16 slices
1 stick (1/2 cup) butter
1 tablespoon garlic salt

Scan the ingredients closely and you will see a lot of fat and a lot of sodium, not to mention a whole lot of calories! Sure, it may taste good if you are used to the taste of high-fat meals, but let's look at the ways we can make this recipe taste good and have a lot less fat, sodium, and fewer, but more nutrient-dense, calories.

Let's start with the lasagna. The first ingredient is meat, and a whole lot of it. A pound of ground beef or ground sausage is a lot of meat. You can get plenty of meat flavor without using that much meat in a recipe. If you replace half of that meat with extra vegetables—you notice this ingredient list is pretty short on vegetables—you will get the same amount, just as filling, but a lot less fat. So let's make that half a pound of ground meat instead of a full pound, and let's add 1 cup of freshly diced tomatoes, a cup of chopped bell peppers—green or red, whichever you like. A cup of fresh spinach tastes great in lasagna. Also, how about adding half a cup of sliced mushrooms for a meaty texture, and half a cup of grated carrots for a little sweetness and beta carotene?

Okay, now let's look at that meat again. Do you need to use ground beef? You can, and if you do, it is better to buy the kind that is 95 percent lean, instead of the cheaper but higher fat kind. It may cost a little more, but think how much you are saving when you only have to **buy** half the amount of meat to make your lasagna. You still come out ahead. Or, for an even better option with less fat that tastes great, have your butcher grind up half a pound of turkey breast and use that.

Now, let's consider the egg. Eggs aren't as bad as we once thought and one isn't much fat, but still, two egg whites contain no fat at all and take the space of one full egg, so let's replace that egg with two egg whites instead. As for the creamy cottage cheese, this isn't necessary. That high-fat cottage cheese isn't any better in a recipe than the low-fat or non-fat kind. Or, replace it with low-fat or non-fat ricotta cheese, which has a smoother texture without those curds. You don't need so much Romano cheese for your lasagna either. Let's cut that down to half a cup, and buy the part-skim mozzarella. Part-skim mozzarella is easy to find in the store; you can cut that in half too, using four ounces instead of eight.

With less meat and cheese, you will want to make the herbs and spices more intense to boost flavor. You've already got a good start with the extra flavors from added vegetables, but greater amounts of herbs and spices will make your lasagna even more substantial and satisfying. Instead of that one tablespoon of Italian seasoning, let's add one tablespoon basil, one teaspoon oregano, one-half teaspoon thyme, and a bay leaf or two. Or consider these variations:

- For a Greek flavor, try adding one-half teaspoon cinnamon and one-fourth teaspoon nutmeg to the sauce.
- For a deeper, smokier flavor add two teaspoons of cumin and a teaspoon of chili powder.
- For a fresh, interesting flavor, try two teaspoons of tarragon.
- How about adding a handful of chopped fresh cilantro to give your lasagna a Mexican kick? Hey, fusion cooking—the blending of different

cuisines like Italian and Mexican—can be lots of fun and can open your mind, and your taste buds, to all kinds of new ideas and flavors.

Half the fun of cooking is experimenting with your herbs and spices. Let the food artist in you come out! Okay, let's see what our low-fat, low-sodium, nutrient-dense Menu for Life recipe looks like:

Healthful Menu for Life Lasagna

Serves 8

1/2 pound extra lean ground beef or ground turkey breast
1 large onion, chopped
1 clove garlic, minced
1 cup of freshly diced tomatoes
1 cup chopped bell peppers
1 cup fresh spinach, finely chopped
1/2 cup sliced mushrooms
1/2 cup of grated carrots
1 8-oz. can tomato sauce, no sodium added
1 6-oz. can tomato paste
1 tablespoon basil
1 teaspoon oregano
1/2 teaspoon thyme
2 bay leaves
1 cup water
6 dried lasagna noodles
2 egg whites, lightly beaten
16-oz. carton non-fat cottage or ricotta cheese
2 tablespoons reduced-sodium grated Romano cheese
4 oz. shredded part-skim mozzarella cheese
2 tablespoons snipped fresh parsley or cilantro for the top
   (or 2 teaspoons dried)

METHOD

1. Preheat oven to 375° F. Spray a 2-qt. casserole or rectangular glass or nonstick baking pan with nonstick cooking spray.
2. In a medium nonstick skillet sprayed with nonstick cooking spray, brown the extra lean ground beef or ground turkey over medium heat until no pink remains in meat, about 10 minutes. Instead of adding the other ingredients at this point, first drain the meat into a colander and rinse lightly with water from sink. This technique can reduce the meat's fat content even more.
3. Spray the pan again with nonstick cooking spray and return the rinsed meat to the pan. Add onions, garlic, fresh tomatoes, bell peppers, spinach, mushrooms, and carrots. Toss with meat, cooking over medium heat until onions are translucent, about 7–8 minutes. Stir in tomato sauce, tomato paste, basil, oregano, thyme, bay leaves, and about a cup of water. Turn heat to medium-high and bring mixture to a boil. Reduce heat, cover, and simmer for about 15 minutes.
4. While sauce is simmering, cook lasagna noodles according to the package directions. Drain, rinse, and drain again. Set aside.
5. To make the cheese filling, mix the egg whites, non-fat cottage or ricotta cheese, and Romano cheese.
6. In the casserole or pan, layer half the noodles, spread with half the cheese filling, followed by half the meat sauce, half the mozzarella cheese, then repeat all the layers. Sprinkle the top with dried or snipped fresh parsley or cilantro.
7. Bake for 30 minutes or until all the layers are hot. Let stand 10 minutes out of the oven, then cut the lasagna into 8 servings.

For your garlic bread, who needs all that butter and sodium? It is the garlic flavor, pungent and sharp, and the bread's texture that make this dish special. Try this healthy update to complement your newer, fresher lasagna. It leaves out the butter but has that buttery flavor you want to taste, authentic olive oil, and more garlic to give this bread lots of intensity. You can bake it in the oven along with the lasagna, on the lower rack.

Healthful Menu for Life Garlic Bread

Serves 8

1 loaf of Italian bread cut into 16 slices
nonstick butter-flavored cooking spray
2 tablespoons extra virgin olive oil
8 cloves garlic, peeled and minced

METHOD:
1. Preheat oven to 375° F.
2. Spray a cookie sheet with nonstick butter-flavored cooking spray.
3. Spread the bread slices on the cookie sheet. Spray lightly with butter-flavored cooking spray.
4. Brush a tiny bit of olive oil on each bread slice with a cooking brush, topped with approximately 1/2 minced garlic clove per slice.
5. Bake until garlic bread and garlic look golden brown, about 15–20 minutes.

See how you can change only a few key things to make the recipes you love just fine to eat when you are trying to get healthy? You *can* do it! And don't think you have to stop with lasagna and garlic bread. You can do all kinds of things to change your favorite recipes into healthful Menu for Life creations. Hit or miss, you will learn a lot along the way and, over time, your successes will establish you among friends and family as a healthful Menu for Life food artist extraordinaire!

General Index

~~~~~~~~~

A separate Recipe Index begins on page 303.

mistaken ideas about, 10–11, 13, 96
morbid, 91
mortality rates and, 14–15, 91
overeating and, *see* overeating
reduction in, in Obesity Study, 47
self-love and, 37
see also weight gain
Obesity Study, 16–17, 44–49
hypothesis in, 44
Obesity Study participants, 17–18
Alquietta Brown, 18, 46, 71, 103, 118,
170
Cedric Williams, 17, 27–28, 34, 50, 90,
92–93, 111, 141
Clarence White, 18, 58, 101, 120,
166
Howard Copeland, 18, 55, 89, 134,
135, 136–37, 171
Marie Primas-Bradshaw, 18, 32, 33, 52,
72, 88, 123, 134, 147, 155–57
Stephanie Dove, 17–18, 32, 34, 37, 99,
101, 107, 137, 170
oils, 157, 177, 178
cooking sprays, 206–7
see also fat, dietary
omega 3 fatty acids, 208, 209
osteoarthritis, 86, 96
movement and, 146
overeating, 20–39
changing times and, 23–24
in cycle of obesity, 32–34, 37
emotional, 32–33, 72, 83, 148, 151,
155, 187
habits of, questionnaire on, 34–36
reasons for, 22, 26, 32, 34–36, 66

pain:
aches and discomfort, 86–87, 132, 146
from exercise, 146
pantothenic acid, 163
parties, 170–71
pasta, 154–55, 156, 160, 177, 217
shopping for, 210–11
phosphorus, 165
physical activity, *see* exercise and physical
activity
pies, 212
pizzas, 216–17

pork, buying, 207
portion sizes, 78–81, 84, 155
serving sizes and, 81–83, 167
potassium, 164, 165
poultry, 177, 178–79
buying, 207–8
nutrient density of, 156
Primas-Bradshaw, Marie, 18, 32, 33, 52,
72, 88, 123, 134, 147, 155–57
processed, prepared, and convenience
foods, 24, 26–27, 153, 154–55, 160,
166
buying, 208, 216–18
carbohydrates hidden in, 158
diet, 172–73
in food journal, 187–89
vegetables, 164
prostate cancer, 106
protein, 70, 159–60, 177, 178
amino acids and, 51, 117–18, 159,
160
caloric value of, 69
as energy source, 115, 117–18
fat and, 160
in food exchanges, 179, 183
food journal and, 187
in Menu for Life Meal Planner, 176,
179, 183, 189
percentage of daily calories from, 50,
51, 176
pyridoxine, 163

Recommended Dietary Allowance
(RDA), 154, 178
restaurants, 155, 170
fast-food, 13, 24, 28, 56, 149–50, 160,
174, 189
riboflavin, 162
rice, 70, 156, 177, 211

salad bars, 214
salads, 213–15
salmon, 208
salt, *see* sodium and salt
Satcher, David, 14
seasonings and spices, 215–16
selenium, 165
self-love, 37, 42

Recipe Index

~~~~~~~~

fruits, *continued*
  baby spinach salad with almonds,
    mandarin oranges, and raspberry-
    lemonade vinaigrette, 222–23
  chai-spiced peach mousse, 270–71
  fresh berry country waffles, 269–70
  pear tofu cheesecake amandine,
    274–75
  sweet-tart fruit salad, 227–28

garlic bread, 288, 292

herb and spice substitutions, 277–79
herb garden dip, 228–29
honey peach vinaigrette, 224–25

jalapeno lime vinaigrette, 225–26

lasagna, 288–91
lemon-butter broccoli florets, 265–66
lime jalapeno vinaigrette, 225–26

main dishes:
  baked stuffed pork loin, 248–50
  barbecue pulled pork sandwiches,
    250–51
  broiled citrus swordfish with Caribbean
    chutney, 240–42
  cold fresh vegetable pizza, 238–39
  green-chili chicken casserole, 260–61
  honey smoked chicken, 256–57
  lasagna, 288–91
  marinated beef strips with orange
    brandy sauce, 254–56
  mustard chicken with collard greens,
    259–60
  nutty chicken stir-fry, 257–59
  oven-fried Cajun catfish, 244–46
  potato sausage pie, 246–47
  reducing fat, sodium, and calories in,
    285–86
  spaghetti with pesto sauce, 230–31
  spicy scallop roll, 242–43
  vegetable pork stir-fry medley,
    252–54
  vegetarian chili, 234–36
meats:
  baked stuffed pork loin, 248–50

barbecue pulled pork sandwiches,
  250–51
marinated beef strips with orange
  brandy sauce, 254–56
spices for, 280
substitutions for, 280–82
vegetable pork stir-fry medley, 252–54
mousse, chai-spiced peach, 270–71
muffins, creamy cornbread, 268–69
mustard chicken with collard greens,
  259–60

orange(s):
  brandy sauce, marinated beef strips
    with, 254–56
  mandarin, baby spinach salad with
    almonds, raspberry-lemonade
    vinaigrette and, 222–23

pasta:
  lasagna, 288–91
  spaghetti with pesto sauce, 230–31
peach:
  honey vinaigrette, 224–25
  mousse, chai-spiced, 270–71
pear tofu cheesecake amandine, 274–75
pepper dressing, cheesy, 226–27
pesto sauce, spaghetti with, 230–31
pie, potato sausage, 246–47
pizza, cold fresh vegetable, 238–39
pork:
  barbecue pulled, sandwiches, 250–51
  loin, baked stuffed, 248–50
  vegetable stir-fry medley, 252–54
potato(es):
  better-than-fried, 263–64
  sausage pie, 246–47
poultry:
  green-chili chicken casserole, 260–61
  honey smoked chicken, 256–57
  mustard chicken with collard greens,
    259–60
  nutty chicken stir-fry, 257–59
  potato sausage pie, 246–47
  spices for, 280
  substitutions for, 280–82